T0216558

Obesity Medicine Made Easy

Obesity is a complex disease, and this brief resource offers a comprehensive review of the most recent evidence on the multitude of ways to help treat this condition. Practically oriented for the reader to understand and easily apply the knowledge to patients, it specifically focuses on the lifestyle medicine approach to obesity management. This means applying the science of nutrition, movement, sleep, and stress with the help of cognitive behavioral therapy, motivational interviewing skills, positive psychology, and the circadian rhythm. This approach is combined with information on anti-obesity medications and bariatric surgery in a concise manner, immensely useful for the busy clinician.

Key Features

- Captures the attention of the readers through a concise, lucid style of text and its organization.
- Offers clarity on a common yet complex topic to physicians, dieticians, nurse practitioners, and healthcare providers, leading to a change in practice and helping patients improve their weight which would impact underlying medical conditions.
- Includes a comprehensive approach to management which combines the importance of medication, lifestyle habits, and behavioral change.

Made Easy

Endocrinology for the Small Animal Practitioner
David Panciera and Anthony Carr

ECG for the Small Animal Practitioner
Larry Tilley and Naomi Burtnick

Obesity Medicine Made Easy
Ananda Chatterjee

Obesity Medicine
Made Easy

Ananda Chatterjee, MD

Foreword by
Holly F. Lofton, MD

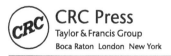

CRC Press
Taylor & Francis Group
Boca Raton London New York

CRC Press is an imprint of the
Taylor & Francis Group, an **informa** business

Designed cover image: Shutterstock

First edition published 2024
by CRC Press
6000 Broken Sound Parkway NW, Suite 300, Boca Raton, FL 33487-2742

and by CRC Press
4 Park Square, Milton Park, Abingdon, Oxon, OX14 4RN

CRC Press is an imprint of Taylor & Francis Group, LLC

© 2024 Ananda Chatterjee

ISBN: 9781032443225 (hbk)
ISBN: 9781032443218 (pbk)
ISBN: 9781003371595 (ebk)

DOI: 10.1201/9781003371595

Typeset in Sabon
by codeMantra

I dedicate this book to my parents. Their sacrifice, dedication, and discipline have led me to this point. All traits I pride myself in now but do not take for granted.

Contents

Foreword by Dr. Holly F. Lofton, MD

'Journey' is often the term used to describe a person's process of weight loss. This is indeed an appropriate term as weight loss attempts are full of trial and error, best intentions, joy, tears, surprises, planning, and contemplation of next steps. Our patients rely on us as partners in this journey, and while we wish we could take every step with them, we are limited to the confines of the duration of our office visits, and meager written or verbal interactions between these visits. Thus, we must make the most of this time as our patients view us as wizards offering pearls of knowledge and support throughout their journey.

As a board-certified obesity medicine physician, educator, and researcher, I continue to be astonished by the continued prevalence of obesity as a disease in our world, despite the tireless energy of providers, such as myself and Dr. Ananda Chatterjee. Obesity is expected to affect 49.2% of Americans and 1 billion people globally by 2030 (1,2). Obesity is a chronic, progressive, relapsing remitting disease that affects all organ systems. Thus, all providers are treating patients with obesity or the sequelae of obesity. As of December 2022, there are currently 5879 board-certified obesity medicine specialists in the United States – certainly too few to treat the 240 million American adults with overweight and obesity (3,4). We need your help! Only 2% of patients eligible for treatment of weight conditions are receiving treatment. Whether you are a medical student, resident, fellow, attending, researcher, or other interested party, your decision to study this guide, and take its principles with you as you practice, will positively impact the obesity epidemic, but most importantly your individual patients' health and well-being immensely.

I was obliged to have the opportunity to select Dr. Chatterjee as a Clinical Obesity Medicine fellow at NYU Grossman School of Medicine, as was captivated by his plentiful publications in topics related to preventive medicine. During his fellowship, Dr. Ananda Chatterjee followed over 500 patients along their journey, bringing his devotion to the fields of Lifestyle and Obesity Medicine to our busy medical weight management practice housed in an urban academic medical center. As the director of the program for over 10 years, I welcomed Dr. Chatterjee's kind and pleasant demeanor. Patients and staff alike praised his thoughtful recommendations both with regard to lifestyle modifications, and medical management of obesity and overweight. After moving on to his own private practice, our patients at NYU continue to thrive based on his efforts. I whole-heartedly support Dr. Chatterjee's contribution to the field of obesity medicine in penning this vital guide to understanding the complex nature of obesity and treating it with both compassion and professional acumen. Prepare to close the cover with a new outlook on the science of obesity and with a new fervor to tackle this disease!

REFERENCES

1. Ward et al. Projected U.S. State-Level Prevalence of Adult Obesity and Severe Obesity. NEJM. 2019; 381:2440–2450.
2. World Obesity Atlas 2022.
3. www.ABOM.org (Accessed December 23, 2022)
4. www.cdc.org/nchs/fastats/obesity-overweight.htm (Accessed December 23, 2022)

Preface

Being a jack of all trades and a master of none is the modus operandi for a primary care physician. For medical specialists in endocrinology, rheumatology, psychiatry, etc. or other allied health professionals (for example dieticians), the opposite is true. They become engrossed in their field of expertise, and that is why we refer to them for specific issues. Either way, making the science of obesity a priority to learn for any of these professionals is not quite there. I am here to argue that if some effort is made in mastering this subject matter, the success and ease at work will amplify and be worth it. This, in turn, will lead to a much happier life overall, in and outside of work.

Every day we health professionals wake up, get ready, and start seeing patients in our busy schedule. We can see patients for acute concerns, chronic medical conditions, or preventative care. Our goals are for patients to not have frequent acute symptoms so that they can enjoy their day-to-day lives better; for chronic medical conditions to be stable and not progress to requiring more medications and specialist visits; and ultimately to avoid dangerous end points such as a cancer diagnosis, hospitalization for severe influenza or COVID-19, suicide or a heart attack. We do our best, based on our knowledge and the brief amount of time we have with the patient. In the end, we rely on the patient to comply with our advice and be adherent to medications, office visits, and living a healthy lifestyle. This puts majority of the onus on the patient. Let's give our patients a fighting chance. Let's give them the knowledge they need. Let's give them the confidence they need. Let's make them accountable and motivate them to be their best self. Otherwise, what are we really doing?

This book will provide information that makes life better for both you and the patient. Sounds pretty good to me. But what will make you even happier is knowing that this information can be applied to patients without sacrificing much time. For 2 years, I practiced family medicine, travel medicine, and obesity medicine in Toronto, Canada. This may sound a bit odd, but on average, I saw 40–70 patients a day. You read that correctly. The health system is different than in the United States, and that volume would not be possible here in the United States. As I saw patients (as if they were coming in on a factory belt line), I did not feel rushed, the patient had all questions answered, AND I was able to apply the skills and knowledge necessary to help my patients change their daily lifestyle habits. Let me explain how.

My medical assistant would ask about stress (on a scale of 1–10), sleep (number of hours slept), exercise (number of minutes per week), and a few nutrition questions and add this information to the vitals. I would quickly glance at the vitals, and if I saw something I could help the patient improve on, I would make a mental note of it. Then, as I saw the patient for a refill of their blood pressure medications or to follow up on their depression, I would weave in a connection to their, for example, poor sleep. I would simply make that connection of sleep to depression or hypertension, and I would ask them just to make sleep a priority. That's all. Maybe I would give some sleep hygiene advice, but my goal was just to encourage them to make sleep a priority and not push it to the side. You never know if that one visit will lead to changes in sleep habits and subsequently improve blood pressure or mood. You just never know but the potential is there. So why not try.

As you read the book and learn about different evidence-based ways to help your patient lose weight, keep in mind that they apply to every medical condition they have. Especially the ones you may care dearly about.

Acknowledgments

I would like to first acknowledge my lovely wife. Without her support I would not have the courage to start a project like this. She is my rock. Next, I would like to thank Dr. Holly Lofton at NYU Langone for her mentorship and kindness. My depth of knowledge in this field is thanks to her.

Author biography

Dr. Ananda Chatterjee is a Family Medicine Physician who is triple board certified in Family Medicine, Obesity Medicine, and Lifestyle Medicine. He has also completed a Fellowship in Obesity Medicine at the NYU Langone School of Medicine. His deep understanding and compassion for patients with obesity has led to a successful private practice in Portland, Oregon. Before that, he was in Toronto, Canada, where his passion of obesity medicine was founded while practicing primary care and travel medicine. He has a deep understanding of the clinical guideline development process and what other physicians desire when looking for educational material. He has published in this realm of knowledge translation, including an article in the *Canadian Medical Association Journal* (*CMAJ*) titled 'How can Canadian guideline recommendations be tested?'. In his spare time, his interests include world travel, fine dining, watching NBA, and the latest binge-worthy TV show.

Chapter 1

Where are we now

Over the last 35 years, the prevalence of obesity has doubled world-wide. That is a very short time for such a large change to occur. In 2014, 11% of men and 15% of women across the globe had obesity.[1] When including people who are overweight (Body Mass Index over 25), this includes 1.9 billion people. The actual estimate is likely more as the definition of overweight is different based on ethnicity. Chronic disease risk occurs with lower BMIs in a large segment of the population (Asian population for example). This disease is not sparing our children either. Over 42 million children under the age of five were overweight or had obesity in 2013.[2] A pandemic is at hand.

It is interesting to note that for most of the 20th century, the rate of obesity in the United States was around 10%. It then linearly progressed from the 1970s and is now approaching 45% today. If we include the overweight category, then this number reaches over 70%. Think about that number. Seven out of ten American adults are overweight. The trend is not looking good either. By 2030, the estimates are that obesity will surpass 50% of the population in the United States.[3]

The story is not that much better for the neighboring countries. In 2018, 26.8% of Canadians 18 and older (roughly 7.3 million adults) were reported to have obesity. Another 9.9 million adults (36.3%) were classified as overweight. Thus, the total population in Canada with increased health risks due to excess weight is 63.1% in 2018. Breaking it down by provinces, the rate of obesity was lowest in the province of British Columbia (23.1) and highest in Newfoundland and Labrador (40.2%). The province of Ontario, which is home to the largest city in Canada (Toronto) had an obesity rate the same as the national average (26.1%).[4] While in Mexico,

DOI: 10.1201/9781003371595-1

the adult rate of obesity was 36.1%. An ominous statistic is that central obesity (waist circumference more than 94 cm in men and 80 cm in women) was prevalent in 81.6% of all adults in Mexico.[5] As we will learn later, waist circumference is a strong indicator of risk for chronic diseases, independent of the BMI. That means eight out of ten adults in Mexico have health risks due to excess fat in the body. These are staggering numbers.

Now Europe has many fundamental practices and governmental regulations that make it more likely for the population to be at a healthy weight, but even they are not spared from the overall trends. Nearly two-thirds (60%) of adults and a third of children in the European region are overweight or have obesity, and no state is on track to meet the target of halting the increase in the prevalence of obesity by 2025, according to a World Health Organization (WHO) statement. Consistent increases in the prevalence of overweight and obesity have been seen across the European region of 53 countries, and early studies indicate that the situation has worsened during the COVID-19 pandemic. Estimates indicate that obesity in the region rose by 21% in the 10 years to 2016 and by 138% since 1975.[6]

The story is a little more complex in the Asia-Pacific region where urbanization and socio-economic status play a distinct and unique role. Adding to the complexity is the lack of data in many regions as well. In most of the Asian countries, the prevalence of overweight and obesity has increased many folds in the past few decades. But wide differences exist in its prevalence. The countries and regions in Asia are at different phases of development. Some like Vietnam and Indonesia are in the early stages of development, while others like Japan, Singapore, Malaysia, and Hong Kong are at more advanced stages. Many Asian countries have rates that are not very different from that in the United States. The highest rate of obesity in Asia is in Thailand, and the lowest is in India followed by the Philippines. China, which once had the leanest of populations, is now rapidly catching up with the West in terms of prevalence of overweight and obesity.[7]

In Singapore, which is a developed region in Asia, nearly 35% of people aged 18–69 years are overweight, and another 14% have obesity. This societal problem in Singapore is shown to be associated with its extremely large GDP and economic affluence. An example of an Asian country with both undernutrition and overnutrition paradox is the Philippines. Among adults, the prevalence of underweight was 13.2%, while the prevalence of overweight was 20.2%.

In a systematic review by Dinsa et al. in 2012,[8] the key findings were that in low-income countries, obesity is more profound in the rich than the poor. However, in middle-income countries, the evidence is mixed. A trend that is found in all countries is that affluent women are more likely to be at a healthy weight than lower socioeconomic status women. Urbanization adds to this complexity. In a systematic review and meta-analysis, they found a consistent positive association between urbanicity and obesity in countries of Southeast Asia, in all age groups and both genders. This association between urbanicity and obesity was greater in lower income countries.[9]

The data is a bit scarce in the Middle East, North Africa, and the sub-Saharan African region. But trends follow the socio-economic and urbanicity themes. For example, in 2008, the average BMI among men in the Democratic Republic of the Congo was 19.9— the lowest in the world. Yet in South Africa, men had an average BMI of 26.9, on par with the average BMIs in Canada (27.5) and the United States (28.5).[10]

Since the 1940s, the mantra of 'Eat Less, Move More' has existed.[11] Where has that got us? Saying the same thing and expecting a different result is the very definition of insanity. Yet, most physicians think that is the answer. Think of eating less calories and moving more as the small tightly bound nucleus of the solution to obesity. In the periphery lies everything else needed for success that is sustainable and enjoyable. This includes other aspects of nutrition such as quality of food and food timing, connecting sleep and stress to obesity, working on cognitive behavioral strategies, and encouraging a positive attitude in your patient. All of this can be accomplished by physicians from all disciplines. But the first major hurdle is us. Our negative attitudes toward obesity and our lack of knowledge.[12]

In 2013, the American Medical Association (AMA) declared obesity a disease. This was a giant step in the right direction. But this concept has not trickled down to most health providers unfortunately. In a 2015 study by King et al.,[13] in 300 hospitalized children, obesity was documented in 8.3% of charts and was addressed in 4%. There are many similar studies. This only happens because of the unfamiliarity of providers to the disease of obesity. A systematic review by Mastrocola in 2020[14] concluded that there is a paucity of obesity medicine education for medical students, residents, and fellow physicians in training programs all over the world. The Society of Behavioral Medicine wrote a Call-to-Action paper in 2021 urging medical educators to include obesity medicine training.[15] It can make a difference. Obesity education in medical students increased empathy toward patients with obesity and confidence level in being able to manage obesity.[16] When a provider is confident in treating a medical condition, they are more likely to seek out that diagnosis and provide optimal care. Let that confidence begin now.

CASE STUDY

Meet Martha. She is a 56-year-old white female who presents to the clinic for the first time to meet Dr. Chatterjee. Her BMI is 36 (Class 2 Obesity), and she was recently told she has pre-diabetes and elevated cholesterol levels. Currently she is on no medications except for some allergy medications as needed and some topical steroids for her mild plaque psoriasis. The purpose of this case study, which you will see continued in other chapters, is to help you see how frequent questions from patients are answered and the way a weight loss visit can proceed.

Dr. C: Good morning, Martha. It is a pleasure to meet you. I am Dr. Chatterjee. I am a Family Medicine Physician who is also board certified in Obesity Medicine. How can I help best today?

M: Thank you for seeing me Dr. Chatterjee. I was hoping you could help me lose some weight. I have tried for years with multiple diets. You name it, and I have tried. Nothing seems to work. Recently, I was told my blood sugar is high and my cholesterol levels. That scared me a little, and I was hoping to control them without going on any medications. My mother used to be on several medications, and I saw her struggle. I do not want to end up like that. Is there a weight loss medication that can help lose this weight so I can avoid diabetes?

Dr. C: We will definitely discuss if there is medication that would work well for you. Let me get a better idea of your medical history, weight loss history, and current lifestyle habits and we can go from there. Does that sound ok?

M: Sounds good to me.

Dr. C: Excellent. Now, I have done a thorough review of your medical chart, including the recent lab work. So, we do not have to go over that. Let us start with your weight loss history. What is your highest weight as an adult? And your lowest weight?

M: My current weight of 210 is my highest. My lowest weight was in my early 20s when I was closer to 140.

Dr. C: Over the last year, how has your weight changed?

M: I have for sure gained some weight. About 20–30 lbs.

Dr. C: Any history of weight loss surgery?

M: No.

Dr. C: Any history of using weight loss medications?

M: No.

Dr. C: Now the lifestyle habits. Every day is different, but on a typical day, can you tell me what you eat/drink, starting from when you wake up all the way to bedtime?

M: Sure. I usually have oatmeal with berries and coffee for breakfast. Sometimes I eat eggs and toast with some bacon. Then for lunch.

Dr. C: Sorry to interrupt you. Can you tell me what time you usually have your breakfast?

M: Around 7 am.

Dr. C: Thank you. Please continue.

M: For lunch it can vary. It is usually something from the cafeteria where I work or a nearby store. It can be a sandwich or a salad. Sometimes a slice of pizza. My lunch is usually at 12 pm. Then I have a snack in the middle of the afternoon. A protein bar or some chips. I get home from work at around 6 pm. I have dinner with my husband. Half the time we order food in, and the other half I make food at home. Usually, some sort of meat with pasta or rice or potatoes. And some veggies.

Dr. C: Is that it? Anything after dinner?

M: I can sometimes have some popcorn while watching TV before going to bed.

Dr. C: Around what time do you usually stop having all calories on most days?

M: I would say by 9 pm.

Dr. C: Thank you. Next would be activity level. Now I break down activity into sedentary time, aerobic activity, weight training, and leisurely activity. We will talk about each of those in more detail at future visits. But for now, do you do any type of exercise, such as walking?

M: I do not. I walk sometimes but not often.

Dr. C: Now I would like to get an idea of your sedentary time. What this means is, from the time you wake up until you go to bed, all the time you are sitting or lying down. Think about how many hours of the day this could be, including the time at work and at home.

M: Well, I am sitting most of the day for work, and then after I come home, I am relaxing. I do the household chores of course. So, I am up and moving then.

Dr. C: Ok, so let's get a rough idea of how many hours daily of sedentary time. What time do you go to bed usually and when do you wake up?

M: I go to bed by midnight, and I wake up by 6:30 am most days.

Dr. C: So that is 17 and a half hours a day that you are awake. How many of those hours on average would you say you are sitting or lying down?

M: I would say 14–15 hours. Hard to say.

Dr. C: That is helpful. Thank you. Next, I wanted to ask about sleep. You told me your sleep times. Are they consistent from weekday to weekend? And do you think the quality of sleep is good most days?

M: I think I sleep well. I sleep in on Saturdays. Need to catch up from the stress of the week.

Dr. C: I can understand that for sure. Speaking of stress. That is my next question. On a scale of 1–10, what would you say is your stress level recently?

M: 7–8.

Dr. C: Now on a scale of 1–10, how happy are you? 10 being the happiest.

M: I am happy. I'd say 10.

Dr. C: Love to hear that. That is wonderful. Now a few more specific questions before we can get to the fun part of creating a weight loss plan. Any history of the following? Eating disorders, pancreatitis, family or personal history of thyroid cancers, seizures, uncontrolled blood pressure, heartbeat issues or regular opioid use?

M: None of those.

Dr. C: Perfect. Now I have a better understanding of how I can help you best.

The case will be continued in the next chapter. Just to summarize. It is important to get details on the patient's weight history, lifestyle habits, and contraindications to anti-obesity medications.

NOTES

1 Arroyo-Johnson et al. *Gastroenterology Clinics of North America* (2016). PMID: 27837773/DOI: 10.1016/j.gtc.2016.07.012

2 Yumak et al. *European Guidelines for Obesity Management in Adults* (2015). PMID: 26641646/DOI: 10.1159/000442721

3 Ward et al. *The New England Journal of Medicine* (2019). PMID: 31851800/DOI: 10.1056/NEJMsa1909301

4 Statistics Canada. 2018. https://www150.statcan.gc.ca/n1/pub/82–625-x/2019001/article/00005-eng.htm (Accessed November 11th 2022)

5 Barquera et al. *The Lancet Diabetes and Endocrinology* (2020). PMID: 32822599/DOI: 10.1016/S2213–8587(20)30269-2

6 WHO European Regional Obesity Report (2022). World Health Organization. https://apps.who.int/iris/handle/10665/353747 (Accessed November 21st 2022)

7 Ramachandran et al. *Journal of Obesity* (2010). PMID: 20871654

8 Dinsa et al. *Obesity Reviews* (2012). PMID: 22764734

9 Angkurawaranon et al. *PLoS One* (2014). PMID: 25426942

10 Finucane et al. *Lancet* (2011). PMID: 21295846

11 Nicholson. *Obesity Medicine Association Conference* (2018)

12 Sebiany et al. *Journal of Family and Community Medicine* (2013). PMID: 24672270

13 King et al. *The Journal of Pediatrics* (2015). PMID: 26254834

14 Mastrocola et al. *International Journal of Obesity* (2020). PMID: 31551484

15 Ockene et al. *Translational Behavioral Medicine* (2021). PMID: 32242625

16 Kushner et al. *BMC Medical Education* (2014). PMID: 24636594

Chapter 2

Why we should care

We are healthcare providers because there is a part of us that wants to see our patients live a long, healthy, and happy life. We become interested in certain aspects of medicine and wellness, and this leads us to our expert knowledge in specialties such as a rheumatology, psychiatry, nutrition, neurology, etc. We become focused on the diseases we see often in our practice and everything else we leave to experts in their respective fields, and rightfully so. When a psychiatrist sees a patient and the patient mentions a painful wrist, the psychiatrist may tell the patient to go see their primary care doctor. Similarly, when an oncologist is seeing a patient with cancer and the patient mentions they are depressed, they will be referred to counseling and a psychiatrist. These are reasonable referrals. Even if you have the knowledge to treat each of these conditions, who has the time to treat cancer, solve a patient's joint pain, and deal with their depression in a 15- to 30-minute office visit? Not very practical. But there is something most healthcare providers can do that takes very little time and can benefit the patient. Let the patient know the different symptoms and conditions they are experiencing are likely related. This would be surprising news to the patient. For example, inflammation is one of the hallmarks of cancer.[1] Inflammation is also inter-related to depression,[2] and we all know about the inflammation that occurs in areas of pain. Thus, inflammation connects these different and seemingly unrelated disease states. To complicate it even further, depression itself can lead to higher mortality rates in cancer patients.[3] If the patient was told by their psychiatrist, oncologist and primary care physician that these conditions are connected, it could help the patient focus on common treatment pathways such as working on healthy lifestyle habits to reduce this inflammation. The challenge for us

DOI: 10.1201/9781003371595-2

healthcare providers is to remember to let the patient know they are connected. We may not know the exact mechanisms behind it, but we can appreciate the relationship. We would benefit from doing this as well. This is because when the patient starts working harder to improve their general health because they now understand it will improve multiple symptoms they are dealing with, the specific medical condition they see you for will likely improve and your job becomes easier. Just like inflammation, think of obesity as part of this underlying thread.

To live longer means avoiding the top ten causes of death. They include in descending order heart disease, cancer, lung disease, accidents, stroke, Alzheimer's dementia, diabetes, influenza/pneumonia, kidney disease, and suicide.[4] All these medical conditions can be connected by common pathological processes. Suicide/depression may not seem related to heart disease, and dementia may not seem connected to diabetes, but they are. Even COVID-19, which entered the top ten causes of death recently, does not escape this fact. In a systematic review and meta-analysis by Ho et al.,[5] obesity led to more severe disease and death. So, what connects all the above? It brings us back to inflammation in the body and a weakened immune system that connects them all together. Obesity worsens both inflammation and the immune system.[6] Hence, no matter what your specialty is, it is very likely that the disease processes you care about are impacted by obesity.

NOTES

1 Hanahan et al. *Cell* (2011). PMID: 21376230
2 Kiecolt-Glaser et al. *The American Journal of Psychiatry* (2015). PMID: 26357876
3 Pinquart et al. *Psychological Medicine* (2010). PMID: 20085667
4 Centers for Disease Control and Prevention. https://www.cdc.gov/nchs/fastats/leading-causes-of-death.htm (Accessed November 21, 2022)
5 Ho et al. *Annals of the Academy of Medicine* (2020). PMID: 33463658
6 de Heredia et al. *The Proceedings of the Nutrition Society* (2012). PMID: 22429824

Chapter 3

What we need to understand

DEFINING OBESITY

Think of obesity as excess weight that is biologically active and generating harmful substances (adipokines and hormones) on a consistent basis that perpetuates obesity and leads to other comorbid conditions.

We use the very crude measurement of BMI to diagnose obesity. Think of BMI as the starting point to estimate risk and then adding to that risk assessment with other measurements such as waist circumference, body fat percentage, and labs. BMI over 25 is pre-obesity or overweight. BMI over 30 is obesity. In Asians, remember to use BMI cut off around 23 for pre-obesity and BMI over 27 as obesity. Waist circumference over 40 inches in white men and 35 inches in white women is correlated with increased heart disease risk and is a better predictor of heart attacks than BMI. In all other ethnicities, risk starts with waist circumference of 35 inches in men and 31 inches in women. For body fat percentage and specifically visceral fat, the gold standard is MRI (no one does that), but you can recommend patients get a DEXA or bioimpedance scan. For men, the risk increases when body fat percentage is over 25% and for women over 32%.

DOI: 10.1201/9781003371595-3

METABOLICALLY HEALTHY
OBESITY IS A MISNOMER

There is a concept that argues that patients with obesity but have no clinical findings of dyslipidemia, abnormal blood sugars, and hypertension are metabolically healthy. As such, a patient with a BMI over 30 may come to see you for their annual physical, get labs done, and the labs all come back normal. You message the patient and tell them everything looks good and see them in a year. Unfortunately, the risk of type 2 diabetes and cardiovascular disease is higher in 'healthy' patients with obesity as compared to healthy lean individuals.[1] This makes perfect sense. Inflammation and reduced immune system functioning from excess body fat leads to damage in the body that standard testing does not pick up. Endothelial dysfunction, heart muscle damage, plaque buildup, rising insulin levels, DNA damage, poor antioxidant levels, etc. are abnormal findings that continuously insult the body. This is a sub-clinical disease. This is what we should be focused on. Sadly, our focus (and that of our patients as well) begins when a patient has had a heart attack or the Hgb A1c has creeped past 6.5. We can do better.

PATHOPHYSIOLOGY

The average yearly weight gain in adults in the United States is only 1–3 lbs a year despite the average caloric intake of 900,000 calories per year. This tells us that the human body is efficient at what it does and has mechanisms in place to regulate weight. The first concept that is crucial to understand is that the physiology of weight regulation is different between lean individuals and individuals with obesity. To add another layer to this, the physiology of weight regulation is different when losing weight versus when trying to maintain the lost weight. Therefore, for the last several decades, the likelihood of losing and sustaining greater than 10% of initial body weight has remained at about 15%.[2]

Think of weight regulation as controlled by three different parts of the brain. There is the 'homeostatic' brain, the 'emotional' brain, and the 'cognitive' brain. The 'homeostatic' brain (mostly located in the hypothalamus) can slow down metabolism and make you hungry (neurons called NPY/AGrP) OR rev up metabolism and help you feel satiated (neurons called POMC/CART).[3] The yin and yang of weight control. Obesity partly occurs because the 'I feel hungry' part of the brain overtakes the 'I feel full' one. This seesaw battle in the brain is won depending on the inputs received by the brain. So, what are these inputs? Chemical messengers or hormones coming from the stomach (ghrelin, the only hormone in the body that makes you hungry), small intestine (CCK, GLP1, PYY), large intestine (GLP1, PYY), adipose tissue (leptin, adiponectin), pancreas (insulin, amylin), and muscles (myokines). Also, nutrients like amino acids, fatty acids, and glucose can enter the brain and influence weight control. Another input that the scientific community is learning more about is the gut microbiome. 'Good' gut bacteria signal the brain through intermediaries to burn fat and increase satiety, while 'bad' gut bacteria do the opposite.[4] As weight gain continues to occur, the 'I feel hungry' side of the hypothalamus gets stronger and the 'I feel full' side gets weaker. Not ideal to say the least. Medications like GLP1 agonists and bupropion directly target this part of the brain to help sway it in the direction for weight loss. This works well to an extent because this is just one aspect of the disease of obesity. It would be naive to think that a medication or any treatment with a single mechanism of action can treat a complex disease. Just like thinking a blood pressure medication on its own can control the complexity of hypertension.

To add to this complexity in obesity, we now consider the 'emotional' brain and 'cognitive' brain. Anger, sadness, loneliness, boredom, hopelessness, anxiety, depression, and stress all lead to changes in the dopamine pathway in the brain (amygdala, ventral striatum, orbitofrontal cortex) that create cravings for 'comfort' foods. This is a separate and distinct mechanism than the hunger from the 'homeostatic' part of the brain. You can now see how everyday life and the emotional rollercoaster that comes with it can override the basic metabolism of the brain that wants to properly regulate calories in and calories out.

When it comes to making decisions about food, which we do over 200 times a day,[5] the patient with obesity is again fighting an uphill battle compared to the lean person. In a meta-analysis looking at 72 studies, it was found that participants with obesity showed broad impairments on executive function, including on tasks primarily utilizing inhibition, cognitive flexibility, working memory, decision-making, verbal fluency, and planning.[6] All skills needed to successfully lose and keep off weight. No wonder this is difficult.

One more concept that is important to understand. As weight loss occurs, the body begins to fight to gain weight back. The dysregulation in the brain described above intensifies. This leads to slower metabolism.[7] But an even more significant change is that the muscles in the body become more efficient and so the same activity level leads to less calories burned.[8] All these changes with weight loss are called metabolic adaptations and roughly add 300–400 calories a day to the total daily energy expenditure. Hence, maintaining weight loss is more difficult than losing weight.

Appreciating these differences in energy metabolism is fundamental to you being able to show empathy to your patient with obesity and you being able to treat obesity in the correct way. This point cannot be emphasized enough. The goal of this section is to understand the complexity of the pathophysiology of obesity and be able to in a simple way explain it to your patient. Your patient does not need to know the finer details, but if you attempt to explain the changes in the body that occurs after weight gain and how those changes make it difficult to lose weight and makes it even more difficult to maintain weight loss, then maybe your patient will stop blaming themselves. If you accomplish this, your patient has a much higher chance of success with your obesity treatment plan. Here is an example of how you may explain this to your patient: 'Obesity is a disease just like high blood pressure or diabetes. Having this disease means your biology is now different compared to people not having the disease. Let me give you an example of how it is different. Suppose there is a plate of freshly made chocolate chip cookies in the waiting room right now. It is way easier for a person who is lean to resist that cookie compared to you and this has nothing to do with your willpower. So do not think you are weak. You are fighting a very powerful disease for which we have no cure. So, what is happening here is that when the cookie smell is in the air, and you see that gooey freshness, your cravings are much higher than in a lean person. Your emotional urge to have that cookie is stronger than in a lean person, and your ability to make a rational decision is compromised. All of this happens because obesity changes the brain and the hormones in the body to make you feel this way because it wants you to keep this weight gain and gain more. Because the body is fighting against your goal of wanting to lose weight, you cannot rely on your willpower. That will never lead to lasting results, and I am sure you are aware of that already as you have been dealing with weight your whole life. Instead, focus on the consistency of healthy lifestyle habits, making changes to your surrounding environment and anti-obesity medications that counter the ill effects of obesity. I hope that made sense.'

CAUSES OF OBESITY

As a healthcare provider, understanding these intrinsic changes and combining them with all the external forces at work to make your patient eat more, move less, disturb their sleep, and make them stressed, gives you an appreciation of the daunting task at hand for your patient.

But this knowledge is what will make you a better healthcare provider. The empathy and kindness you show to your patient because you understand the multitude of reasons why obesity has occurred and persists, will give you a tremendous advantage when it comes to helping your patient be successful at weight loss.

Nonmodifiable

Genetics

Ninety-nine percent of obesity is polygenic with over 700 genes identified to be associated with excess weight. If patients ask, you can say 30%–40% of their obesity is related to several genes in the body that conspire together to make it difficult to lose weight.[9] Any time genetics is discussed, the flip side must be mentioned as well. Remind the patient that the other 60%–70% is related to environmental circumstances and can be worked on. This information is vital for the patient's self-efficacy. In addition to the heritability of weight, energy expenditure, food choices, hunger, satiation, thermic response to food, and spontaneous physical activity are, to a variable degree, heritable as well.[10,11,12] There are monogenic forms of obesity such as leptin deficiency and POMC deficiency, but they are rare.

Prenatal history

Traits of the mother during her pregnancy such as overnutrition, undernutrition, high BMI, and diabetes can influence health and weight of the future child.[13] The mechanism is deeper than the cellular level. The environmental milieu exposed to the fetus by the mother based on her daily habits can lead to epigenetic modifications that can alter gene expression without affecting the DNA sequence. Essential epigenetic mechanisms include histone modifications, non-coding RNAs, and DNA methylation. This fetal programming from the mother that alters epigenetics is more permanent than you think and can remain for decades or the entire lifespan. Research in this area is growing, and the strongest evidence to date are animal studies. Human clinical studies do show influence of the mothers' fetal environment on the future offspring, but larger studies are needed.[14]

Childhood

Higher weight in childhood influences weight as an adult.[15] The impact excess weight has on a child can be everlasting. It reduces their quality-of-life right from a young age. The psychosocial complications of obesity include depression, body dissatisfaction, unhealthy weight control behaviors, stigmatization, and poor self-esteem.[16] In cognitive behavioral therapy, an important topic is core beliefs. Core beliefs in patients with obesity are deep underpinnings of why a patient has a certain reaction or relationship to food. These core beliefs start in childhood. In addition, this period of life is where habits and cultural aspects from family are ingrained. As such, when patients with obesity mention that obesity runs in the family, it is important to make a distinction between genetic contributions from the parent and contributions from shared habits. Highlighting this salient point to your patient will help put the weight loss effort more in their control and boost their self-efficacy.

Modifiable

Epigenetics

One of the best-studied epigenetic mechanisms is DNA methylation. DNA methylation is defined as the addition of a methyl group to cytosine and is carried out by DNA methyltransferases. In general, hypomethylation of promoter regions leads to an increased expression of a respective gene (turning on a gene), whereas hypermethylation results in transcriptional repression (turning off a gene).[17] It is radical to think that when you eat certain foods, it may be altering the expression of your genes. That seems not possible. But it is happening. Healthy foods eaten on a consistent basis can turn off 'bad' genes and turn on 'good' genes. Similarly, unhealthy foods can do the opposite.

Dr. Dean Ornish is famous for becoming former President of the United States Bill Clinton's doctor after he suffered from a heart attack. The Ornish diet is basically a plant-based, low-fat (10% fat) eating plan that emphasizes avoidance of simple sugars in combination with exercise and stress reduction strategies.[18] In a seminal paper in *JAMA* (*Journal of the American Medical Association*), this specific diet showed it can reverse the diameter of plaque in the coronary arteries.[19] A powerful message that nutrition can influence health. In the GEMINAL (Gene Expression Modulation by Intervention with Nutrition and Lifestyle) study, Dr. Ornish examined changes in prostate gene expression in a unique population of men with low-risk prostate cancer who declined immediate surgery, hormonal therapy, or radiation and participated in an intensive nutrition and lifestyle intervention while undergoing careful surveillance for tumor progression. The results showed that this lifestyle intervention turned on 48 'good' genes and turned off 453 'bad' genes. The conclusion is that intensive nutrition and lifestyle changes may modulate gene expression.[20]

This is important information for your patients. You can tell them that their genetics may be making them prone to obesity, but they have the power to turn off those bad genetics. This puts the patient in the driver's seat. Sometimes that is all that is needed for the patient to get on the right track. A large part of life living with obesity is the helplessness patients feel. It may seem to them that they are destined for it, and so they may not be motivated to make any changes. Give them their control back by offering this powerful information.

Medical conditions

Two conditions most textbooks talk about as a cause for obesity are hypothyroidism and Cushing's syndrome. TSH is part of the labs during assessment, but Cushing's would be rare, and labs ordered only if common physical exam findings are seen such as abdominal purple striae. Another distinguishing aspect of Cushing's is that there is usually accumulation of fat tissue in the face and neck, while sparing the extremities. When it comes to the TSH lab value, if it is slightly above the upper limit of normal, do not assume that the thyroid may be causing the weight gain. It is more likely that the elevated TSH is a marker of obesity.[21] With weight loss, the TSH can return to the normal range.

A medical condition that is far more common and should be on your radar as contributing to obesity is major depressive disorder. There is a bidirectional relationship here as depression leads to a higher risk of obesity and vice versa.[22] Depression can affect quality and quantity of sleep, stress levels, snacking of processed foods at odd times, and less movement throughout the day. There may also be a shared biological pathway linking the two diseases.[23] If you see depression as a comorbid condition, make it a priority to discuss. Healthy habits that can help with weight loss should help with depression as well. Make that connection for the patient.

Food quantity

In the 1970s, food intake was 2,398 kcal/day/person, and this increased to 2,895 kcal/day/person in the 2000s. This increase in energy intake is enough to explain the increase in the prevalence of obesity we have seen.[24] This has happened despite the universal knowledge that eating less is good for weight loss. A part of the reason is all the hidden calories in society today due to increased consumption of processed foods. Food manufacturers are really packing in the calories in food items that look small, such as a cookie. This size or volume of food is important to note as humans are good at judging the amount of food to eat daily and not good at guessing the calories of the foods they consume. Volumetrics is a concept discussed later that tackles this problem.

You will not be introducing a new concept to your patients when you suggest less food. This should lead us to the conclusion that we have to help the patient in other ways. Simply telling our patients to eat less is like telling a patient to swim without any swimming lessons. Good luck with that!

Food quality

All calories are not made equal (Figure 3.1). Let's take, for example, a calorie-dense healthy food such as beans or nuts versus say a chocolate chip muffin. The first concept to understand is that the

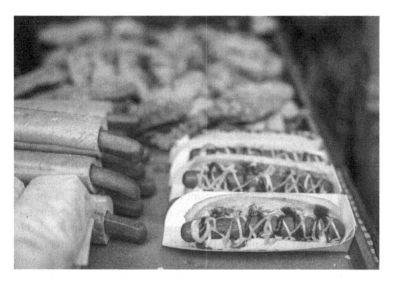

Figure 3.1 One food group you should focus on reducing in your patient's eating habits first is processed meat. This includes sausage, hot dogs, cold cuts, and bacon as common examples. They are considered group 1 carcinogens. They are densely packed with calories. The salt content does not help the weight loss efforts as well.

calories that count are the calories that are *absorbed* by the gut. There is a good percentage of beans and nuts that travel through to the large colon and do not get absorbed by the body due to the fiber content. Second, the fiber in healthy foods like beans or lentils leads to a so-called second meal effect. Dr. David Jenkins in 1981 showed how the glycemic response after consuming a legume like lentils is low.[25] This is good for our patients. But what was fascinating about this study is that having lentils for breakfast caused a lower glycemic response to the foods (such as a piece of bread) eaten at lunch. The benefits of this specific food continued long after its consumption. In contrast, a muffin has a higher glycemic index, which means the blood sugar spike afterward is much higher and can lead to a large drop in blood sugar hours later. This drop in blood sugar leads to a feeling of hunger, and the patient starts looking for food again. Plus, the dopamine response to the muffin leads to craving for calorie-dense unhealthy foods later as well. You can see how slowly changing the quality of a patient's eating habits can lead to better results for weight loss and long-term health overall.

Less movement

Technology has grown at an exponential pace. At almost every turn, there is now a new way of doing things. It seems like most of these new ways allow actions to be completed with ease as compared to before. This is great, but it also has led to engineering out natural movement. Natural movement throughout the day is one of the common elements of the folks that live in the blue zones.[26] The blue zones are areas of the world that have people living over 100 in an atypical amount. Mostly these locations involve a rural setting. In the industrialized world, there are far too many opportunities to sit. As a result, we must plan physical activity and we are not doing a good enough job. Only 23% of the population aged 18–65 meet the current activity standards (150 minutes of moderate-intensity exercise or 75 minutes of high-intensity exercise per week) recommended for general health.[27] In a national study that used accelerometers, 9.6% of adults met the recommended levels of physical activity.[28] Some activity, even if not reaching the recommended guidelines, is better than none. But one-third of adults report zero leisure time activity. The connection of obesity and physical activity is not straightforward, but the main idea is caloric energy expenditure. The total daily energy expenditure (TDEE) is a combination of your basal metabolic rate (the energy you spend just sitting or sleeping), the thermic effect of food (the calories burned while digesting the food you eat), and movement. Movement can be broken down into leisure time activity (like going to the gym) and something called NEAT (non-exercise activity thermogenesis)—a scientific way of saying all movement other than exercise. This includes daily transportation like walking and the activity level at work. From all these different ways to burn calories, movement is the most variable part among different individuals. We can make a big difference by helping the patient engineer activity into their daily routine.

The world sometimes goes through cycles or trends. The fashion industry is known for this. Recently, it seems like technology is helping improve natural movement instead of halting its progress (apps that track steps and home fitness equipment). Let's hope that continues.

Lack of sleep

Short sleep duration (less than 7.5 hours) can occur due to individuals making work, school, or home life a priority. Social habits, whether spending time with friends or playing video games, are another cause for insufficient sleep duration. This is the norm, as cultural tendencies lean to sleep being for the 'weak.' At any given time, 30% of the population may have insomnia symptoms.[29] A meta-analysis found that those with short sleep duration had a 55% higher risk of obesity and that the BMI could be reduced by 0.35 for every hour of sleep increased.[30]

As important as total duration is the quality of sleep. The quality can be affected by sleep hygiene (for example, a glass of wine close to bedtime) and medical conditions that cause physical or mental symptoms. The common concerns include pain control, generalized anxiety disorder, major depressive disorder and obstructive sleep apnea (OSA). OSA has an estimated prevalence of 27%–34% among men 30–70 years of age (9%–28% in women), with a much higher prevalence in patients with obesity.[31] OSA and obesity have a bidirectional relationship and it likely contributes to the inflammation and hormonal changes that perpetuate obesity.[32] Have a high degree of suspicion for this medical condition in your patients with obesity and refer them for a sleep study.

Stress

The stress response is the generalized response to any external stimulus (real or perceived) that has the potential to overwhelm the body's compensatory ability to maintain homeostasis. This response is meant to change the physiology in the body to help us tackle this outside factor (for example, an important project deadline and its stress allow us to focus on the task at hand). In the short term, there is absolutely nothing wrong with that. The problem arises when this response is put in overdrive and continues to change the physiology for an extended period (for example, a job where there is a daunting project deadline every week). In a meta-analysis of longitudinal studies, stress was connected to adiposity, albeit a small effect.[33]

Weight-gaining medications

Medications leading to subtle or overt weight gain is common. Go through your patient's medication list, and see if there are medications that can lead to weight gain. Once identified, see if there is an option to switch to a weight-neutral or weight-negative medication. The common medications to look out for include quetiapine, olanzapine, risperidone, lithium, valproate, gabapentin, pregabalin, amitriptyline, paroxetine, mirtazapine, Depo Provera, glucocorticoids, estrogens, diphenhydramine, insulin, sulfonylureas, thiazolidinediones, and some beta blockers like propranolol and metoprolol.

Governmental policies

Major subsidies to the sugar, grains, and dairy and meat industries have led to the availability of cheap processed foods like cheeseburgers to the masses, while fruits and vegetables undergo minimal subsidization. This trend is portrayed in how Americans eat. Why spend money on spinach and avocados, when you can feed a family of 4 for $15 with value menu items. The economic consequences of obesity and related comorbid conditions such as diabetes are not factored into the equation appropriately. For Canada, the annual societal costs were estimated to be CAD $1.0 billion, according to Krueger et al. in 2015.[34] In Germany, using insurance company data, the estimated costs were 63 billion euros per year.[35] In the United States, the current estimate of $48 billion is predicted to turn into $66 billion by 2030.[36]

Food marketing

Cereal commercials during cartoon shows, the placement of processed foods at eye level in grocery aisles, and the engineering of specific fatty, salty, and sweet taste combinations by scientists working for companies like Nestle or Coca Cola are a few examples of how food marketing works to maximize intake of processed foods (Figure 3.2). This lust for profit has led to the creation of hyperpalatable foods. Hyperpalatable foods are foods with a combination of nutrients (for example, fats mixed with carbs) such as pizza, cookies, crackers, chips, cheeseburgers, and ice cream. Sixty-two percent of all available foods in the United States are hyperpalatable foods.[37] Seventy percent of them are fat/sodium combos, 25% fat and sugar combo, and 16% carb and salt. They take advantage of sensory-specific satiety (the concept that the brain can lose interest in a food if there is one specific nutrient, but when combined with another nutrient or taste, the brain can continue to crave) and lead to food being more enjoyable past the usual 2–3 bites when food typically loses its enjoyment. Highly palatable foods are prepared like a drug would be created. For example, added sugar or salt is stripped to its basic components from natural sugar

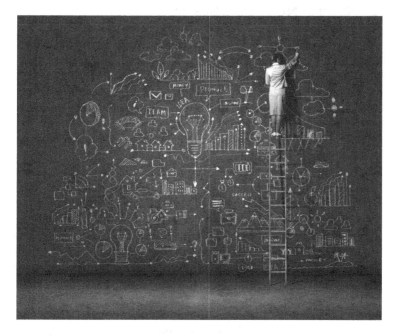

Figure 3.2 Millions of dollars are spent by corporations so that they can entice people onto their food products and get them hooked to have more. They have teams of engineers, marketing experts, food scientists, behavioral scientists, etc. that study the human condition and create super addictive tastes. How can you expect your patient to win this battle on their own?

(the fiber and water) and the concentration is much larger than what is typically found in natural products. In 1988, 49% of foods were hyperpalatable, now in 2018 close to 70%. Fast food, fried items, sweets, and desserts are about 85% of hyperpalatable foods, while fresh fruits, meat, fish, nuts, heavy cream, and vegetables are non-hyperpalatable foods. A key point here is that these foods are made to make you want more, and so suggesting to patients to have them in moderation may not be a good strategy, as by design, these foods are hard to resist.

Global food brands will always look to maximize profits. Some countries are fighting back for the good of society. In 2020, the UK government announced its obesity strategy for England, which included a ban on television and online advertisements for food high in fat, sugar, and salt before 9 pm and an end to 'buy one and get one free' deals on unhealthy food.[38] We must start somewhere.

CONSEQUENCES OF OBESITY

A good way to explain the consequences of obesity is to divide it into immediate effects (for example, diminished cognition, poor concentration, fatigue, mood changes, prone to infections, weight bias), long-term effects (for example, dementia, heart attack, cancers), and the fallout (time wasted at doctors' appointments, cost of medications, hospital visits) from both.

Death would seem to be a good motivator. You can tell your patient that in a meta-analysis including over 30 million individuals, both obesity and overweight were associated with an increased risk of all-cause mortality.[39] The lowest risk was in the BMI range of 20–22. Another study showed that mild obesity equates to loss of 3–4 years of life, while severe obesity leads to loss of 7–8 years when compared to normal-weight individuals.[40] The problem is that these numbers do not speak to your patient. It would be more traumatizing to the patient and a cause for motivation if they found out that the psoriasis patch on their elbow is related to their weight.

There are more than 200 medical conditions associated with obesity. Therefore, it is useful to take an obesity-centric approach when treating these conditions. A good way to organize the common medical conditions associated with obesity is to think of them from head to toe as follows:

Major Depressive Disorder, Generalized Anxiety Disorder, Stroke, Cataracts, Thyroid Disorders, Obstructive Sleep Apnea, Asthma, Chronic Obstructive Pulmonary Disease, Heart Disease, Hypertension, Dyslipidemia, Diabetes, Breast Cancer, Other GI Cancers, Non Alcoholic Fatty Liver Disease, Gastroesophageal Reflux Disease, Gallbladder Disease, Inflammatory Bowel Disease, Irritable Bowel Syndrome, Polycystic Ovarian Syndrome, Low Testosterone, Infertility, Hemorrhoids, Osteoarthritis, Varicose Veins, Gout, Cellulitis, Psoriasis, and Intertrigo.

You can use this list to show patients all the diseases they can avoid and the subsequent cost in terms of time (medical office visits, pharmacy visits, hospital visits) and money (medical office visits, medication costs, hospital visits, etc.). In 2016, the aggregate medical cost due to obesity among adults in the United States was $260.6 billion.[41] On an individual level, adults with obesity in the United States compared with those with normal weight experienced higher annual medical care costs by $2,505 or 100%. The costs increased significantly with class of obesity, from 68.4% for class 1 to 233.6% for class 3.

Another consequence not easily discerned is the effect of obesity on health-related quality of life. In its 1946 Constitution, the World Health Organization defined 'health' as 'a state of complete physical, mental, and social well-being and not merely the absence of disease or infirmity' (WHO. Constitution of the World Health Organization. WHO: Geneva, July 22, 1946). This definition is excellent in highlighting the subtle consequences of obesity outside the obvious comorbid medical conditions. Studies have demonstrated that individuals with obesity experience significant impairments in quality of life, with greater impairments associated with greater degrees of obesity.[42]

WEIGHT BIAS

The Obesity Action Coalition is an excellent resource for patients with obesity and their health providers. Their definition of weight bias is negative attitudes, beliefs, judgments, stereotypes, and discriminatory acts aimed at individuals simply because of their weight. This is a pervasive issue that the patient experiences at home, at work, and in public settings. The media may be the number one culprit (OAC online survey), and another common source of anguish for patients is their own family members (OAC website). The troubling part is that they are subjected to weight bias in the healthcare setting as well. In one study, physicians indicated that they would spend 28% less time with a patient with obesity than they would spend with a patient of normal weight.[43] Other aspects of weight bias in the healthcare setting include chairs in the waiting room that don't fit the patient, the large blood pressure cuff is not available, and the doctor blaming the patient for his/her high blood pressure because he or she is overweight. At this point, you may be wondering that excess weight is the cause of high blood pressure so why is that wrong to mention. Well, it is the way you bring up weight that matters. It is vital to make the connection of excess weight to high blood pressure so patients can be educated and motivated to make changes. But the topic must be brought up with empathy and kindness.

This is crucial not only because it is dehumanizing to experience weight bias but because several studies have shown that weight bias on its own perpetuates obesity and its comorbid conditions. In patients who experience weight stigma, eating increases,[44] self-regulation decreases,[45] their cortisol (an obesogenic hormone) levels are higher, and exercise avoidance is more prominent.[46] We know mental health can affect obesity. Individuals discriminated against based on weight are roughly 2.5 times as likely to experience mood or anxiety disorders.[47] Finally, in a study including 5,079 adults, people who reported experiencing weight discrimination had a 60% increased risk of dying, independent of BMI.[48]

Other examples of weight bias include a patient not going to their doctor because she is afraid of the doctor bringing up weight issues; a patient not going to the gym because she feels ashamed of her body; and a patient feeling depressed because of the way her coworkers look at her and so she overeats unhealthy foods. As you can see, just the stigma of obesity can sabotage a successful weight loss program. All we need to do is acknowledge that the patient sitting in front of you with obesity has experienced weight bias and be kind. You do that and the weight loss program you advocate for has a fighting chance.

CASE STUDY CONTINUED

We completed the patient history and now can discuss the assessment and plan.

Dr. C: Now, I would like to summarize my thoughts on my full assessment and then discuss treatment options. Please feel free to ask me any questions at any time. This entire visit is for your benefit.

M: Thank you.

Dr. C: Your BMI is 36. This is considered class 2 obesity and is a definite risk factor for future chronic diseases. You also have some comorbid conditions of high cholesterol, pre-diabetes, psoriasis, and seasonal allergies. All of these are connected to excess weight and have a chance to improve with some weight loss. More specifically, just 5%–10% weight loss can lower the risk for chronic diseases and improve your current conditions by 50%. That is a powerful motivation to lose that first 5%–10% of weight. Which in our case would be 11–21 lbs. So, 11 lbs would be our first weight loss goal. Does that make sense so far?

M: Yes.

Dr. C: Let me explain very briefly what obesity, the disease, is and what contributes to it. This way you can appreciate why a comprehensive treatment plan is necessary for the best short- and long-term success. And it will also make clear that what we are trying to do here is hard. You know this of course, as you have been dealing with this your whole life.

M: I sure have.

Dr. C: The disease of obesity occurs when there is excess fat. This excess fat accumulates over time and leads to the production of hormones in the body that talk to other parts of the body and the brain. This talk is not friendly as it leads to the body becoming hungrier, craving more, slower metabolism, and makes you insulin resistant. Now when I say insulin resistant, what that means is that when you eat something, instead of 80% or more of it going into the muscles to be used up, it bounces off the muscle and stays in your bloodstream and may end up in the fat cells. So, to summarize, on a daily basis, compared to someone without obesity, you are fighting more hunger, more cravings, and slightly slower metabolism, and when you eat something, it does not get metabolized properly and goes into the fat cells. That is a lot to deal with every single day. It is a vicious cycle that leads to more weight gain. So, my main point here is that this is not your fault. And you cannot compare yourself and what you do on a daily basis to others who are not dealing with obesity. It is a completely different playing field. If I can use a sports terminology.

M: I did not know any of that.

Dr. C: That is ok. That is why you are here today. Now, there is another obstacle to deal with. Your body loves to remember your highest weight. Which currently for you is 210. So, say you reach your first goal of losing 5% of your body weight. 11 lbs of weight loss. At that point, the body does you no favors and changes the hormones in your body to make you even hungrier and slows your metabolism even further. Kind of evil wouldn't you say?

M: Wow.

Dr. C: But the good news is we can make changes to our habits to reduce this hunger. This changing of habits is no easy feat of course. And this is where anti-obesity medications or weight loss surgery helps tremendously. They make it easier for you to accomplish healthy lifestyle habits. Now I have said a lot of new things. Any questions on that?

M: It makes sense. No questions at the moment. I am excited to start this weight loss journey again.

Dr. C: I am too. Let us discuss that plan right now.

NOTES

1   Bluher. *Endocrine Reviews* (2020). PMID: 32128581
2   Kraschnewski et al. *International Journal of Obesity* (2010). PMID: 20479763
3   Valassi et al. *Nutrition, Metabolism and Cardiovascular Diseases* (2008). PMID: 18061414
4   Gupta et al. *Nature Reviews. Gastroenterology and Hepatology* (2020). PMID: 32855515
5   Wansink et al. *Obesity* (2007). PMID: 18198299
6   Yang et al. *Neuroscience and Biobehavioral Reviews* (2018). PMID: 29203421
7   Rosenbaum et al. *Obesity* (2016). PMID: 27460711
8   Goldsmith et al. *American Journal of Physiology* (2010). PMID: 19889869
9   Loos et al. *Current Opinion in Genetics and Development* (2018). PMID: 29529423
10   Perusse et al. *Obesity Research* (2005). PMID: 15833932
11   Llewllyn et al. *Current Obesity Reports* (2017). PMID: 28236287
12   Jiang et al. *PLoS One* (2018). PMID: 30071075
13   Agarwal et al. *Critical Reviews in Clinical Laboratory Sciences* (2018). PMID: 29308692
14   Reichetzeder. *European Journal of Clinical Nutrition* (2021). PMID: 34230629
15   Singh et al. *Obesity Reviews* (2008). PMID: 18331423
16   Vander Wal et al. *Pediatric Clinicas of North America* (2011). PMID: 22093858
17   Jaenisch et al. *Nature Genetics* (2003). PMID: 12610534
18   Ornish. The *New England Journal of Medicine* (2008). PMID: 19009670
19   Ornish et al. *JAMA* (1998). PMID: 9863851
20   Ornish et al. *Proceedings of the National Academy of Sciences of the United States of America* (2008). PMID: 18559852
21   Rotondi et al. *The Journal of Clinical Endocrinology and Metabolism* (2011). PMID: 21296993
22   Luppino et al. *Archives of General Psychiatry* (2010). PMID: 20194822
23   Milaneschi et al. *Molecular Psychiatry* (2019). PMID: 29453413
24   Swinburn et al. *The American Journal of Clinical Nutrition* (2009). PMID: 19369382
25   Jenkins et al. *The American Journal of Clinical Nutrition* (1981). PMID: 6259925
26   Legrand et al. *International Journal of Environmental Research and Public Health* (2021). PMID: 34205297

27 Blackwell et al. CDC National Health Statistics Report (2018). https:// www.cdc.gov/nchs/data/nhsr/nhsr112.pdf (Accessed November 26, 2022)

28 Tucker et al. *American Journal of Preventative Medicine* (2011). PMID: 21406280

29 Ohayon et al. *Sleep Medicine Reviews* (2002). PMID: 12531146

30 Cappuccio et al. *Sleep* (2008). PMID: 18517032

31 Peppard et al. *American Journal of Epidemiology* (2013). PMID: 23589584

32 Jehan et al. *Sleep Medicine and Disorders: International Journal* (2017). PMID: 29517065

33 Wardle et al. *Obesity* (2011). PMID: 20948519

34 Krueger et al. *Canadian Journal of Public Health* (2015). PMID: 26285186

35 Konig et al. *Age and Ageing* (2015). PMID: 25829392

36 Wang et al. *Lancet* (2011). PMID: 21872750

37 Fazzino et al. *Obesity* (2019). PMID: 31689013

38 Mahase. *BMJ* (2020). PMID: 32718928

39 Aune et al. *BMJ* (2016). PMID: 27146380

40 Nyberg et al. *The Lancet: Public Health* (2018). PMID: 30177479

41 Cawley et al. *Journal of Managed Care and Specialty Pharmacy* (2021). PMID: 33470881

42 Kolotkin et al. *Obesity Reviews* (2001). PMID: 12119993

43 Phelan et al. *Obesity Reviews* (2015). PMID: 25752756

44 Schvey et al. *Obesity* (2011). PMID: 21760636

45 Major et al. *Journal of Experimental Social Psychology* (2014). DOI: 10.1016/j.jesp.2013.11.009

46 Vartanian et al. *Journal of Health Psychology* (2008). PMID: 18086724

47 Hatzenbeuhler et al. *Obesity* (2009). PMID: 19390520

48 Sutin et al. *Psychological Science* (2015). PMID: 26420442

Chapter 4

What can we do

Acknowledgment that obesity is a disease is an excellent start. The American Medical Association made that designation in 2013. Then understanding how the physiology of the disease in combination with the environment makes it difficult for patients will give you the empathy needed to connect to your patients. Once that connection is made, the next step is a thorough assessment. Not for a 'cause' of obesity but to look for co-morbidities and clues to the best plan forward. That brings us to the treatment game plan. It includes using cognitive behavioral therapy skills, positive psychology attitudes and motivational interviewing techniques to change lifestyle habits with the help of weight loss medications and/or bariatric surgery.

A general framework that is helpful is the 5 As (Ask, Assess, Advise, Agree, Assist/Arrange). It is popular for helping patients quit smoking. It has been shown in our world of obesity medicine to aid in the communication between a patient and provider in a primary care setting.[1] Just have the general framework in the back of your mind to help structure your thought process. Ask stands for asking for permission to discuss weight. You may not have to do this if you have already tied the patient's excess weight to a specific medical condition that you are addressing at the visit. But it is a polite way to pivot to focus on weight loss. You will be shocked at how appreciative patients can be when they hear you ask if you can discuss their weight. They may start telling you stories of how other providers may have been rude to them in the past and that is why they don't like discussing their weight. Asking for permission is a powerful icebreaker. The second 'A' is Assessment and is what we will discuss briefly in the next section. Based on that assessment, we Advise (the third 'A' in the framework) the patient on the best next steps in terms of changing lifestyle habits, anti-obesity medications and possible bariatric surgery. The fourth 'A' is Agree and is the key step. This is where most providers struggle. Telling a patient to eat less and move more is what we kind of do now. Not very helpful to the patient unfortunately. The skills learned in Chapter 5 will help with this step. This is where realistic and specific goals are made on a task the patient chooses to work on. The final 'A' in the framework is Assist/Arrange for follow-up so that the patient can stay accountable and hopefully reach their goals over time.

ASSESSMENT

The goal here is to confirm if the patient has excess fat, the severity of the condition, look for co-morbidities, find individualized triggers for the weight gain, and determine the patients' motivations and goals.

This assessment can specifically include:

Vitals – blood pressure, heart rate, weight, body mass index, and waist circumference measurement.

Clinical history – general medical history, preventative screening history for cancers, weight history, 24-hour dietary recall for a typical day, hours of sedentary time daily, exercise type/intensity/minutes per week, sleep quantity and quality, stress level on a scale of 1–10, happiness on a scale of 1–10, motivations for weight loss, weight loss goals, screening for sleep apnea using STOPBANG questionnaire, screening for binge-eating disorder (BED) (by asking if they eat more in a 2-hour period, then what most people do on a weekly basis, and during these 2 hours, if they feel out of control), depression screening with PHQ2 and anxiety screening with GAD2.

Diagnostics – body fat% measurement with a body composition machine can be done at a local gym or physical therapy clinic. EKG (if starting a stimulant medication like phentermine), labs (CBC, CMP, TSH, Hgb A1c, lipid panel, apolipoprotein b, lipoprotein (a), insulin, uric acid, hs-CRP, vitamin D, urinalysis; some of these labs may not be considered to be routine or what national guidelines endorse, but our goal is to elicit any subclinical heart disease), FIB4 score (age, AST, ALT and platelet levels to help predict any advanced fibrosis), ASCVD risk calculation, coronary artery calcium (CAC) score, imaging (ultrasound or Fibroscan for fatty liver suspicion) and referrals (common referrals include sleep medicine for a sleep study and gastroenterology for a Fibroscan).

Any abnormality discovered during this assessment, big or small, may be the trigger for change that the patient needs. You never know.

TREATMENT

The heterogeneity of any treatment for most medical conditions is an important concept to always keep in mind. Whether it is intermittent fasting, a low-carbohydrate eating plan, a medication like phentermine or even bariatric surgery; there will be responders and non-responders. This is where personalized medicine becomes important. The entire purpose of a good assessment is to individualize the treatment as best as you can to give the patient the greatest chance of success.

Think of all the below treatment strategies as tools in the tool belt. From all the tools available, most patients may be able to consistently do one-third of them. Our job is to find out which tools these are. Is it eating in an 8-hour window? Is it having a smaller dinner? Is it 10 minutes of aerobic exercise versus 60 minutes? Or is it going to sleep at an earlier time? A patient may be able to do all the above, but we cannot expect our patients to make every change necessary for weight loss to occur. We can, however, figure out what they are willing to try and start there.

Lifestyle interventions

These are the day-to-day habits that can change the physiology of the patient and lead to weight loss and a better cardiometabolic profile. The problem is only 3% of the US population are consistently doing the basic amount needed for good health.[2] The good news is that 97% of the population can benefit from your diligent and persistent advice on this topic.

When to eat

By now everyone has heard of intermittent fasting. What started off as a fad is now mainstream with plenty of science behind it. What does the science say? A systematic review of human trials in overweight/obese subjects that were at least 8 weeks long found intermittent fasting equal to caloric restriction in terms of magnitude of weight loss.[3] There are different types of intermittent fasting.

These include alternate-day fasting (24-hour fast every other day), alternate-day modified fasting (500 calories or less every other day), time-restricted feeding (eating all food in a certain window of time daily), 5:2 fast (5 days of the week you do time-restricted feeding, while the other 2 days you do not) and fasting-mimicking diet (plant based, low protein and 1,000 calories day 1 and 700 calories or less from day 2 through 5; the 5-day fast is done periodically, say every 3 months). Most people who try to do intermittent fasting do time-restricted feeding, with 16 hours of fasting and 8 hours of eating the common pattern. The most popular times that fit most people's schedule is 12 pm to 8 pm. The evidence is showing that time-restricted feeding leads to 20% less caloric intake, reduces body weight and fat mass,[4,5] reduces inflammation, activates brown adipose tissue,[6] reduces hepatic glucose production, decreases hunger, reduces glucose and insulin levels, increases fat burning, lowers blood pressure, reduces oxidative stress, and improves sleep and energy levels,[7,8,9] just to name a few findings. When we dive further into the details, it looks like completing the eating window earlier is better than later.[10,11,12] This means eating from 8 am to 4 pm may be better than 12 pm to 8 pm. This goes hand in hand with the notion that breakfast is important for weight loss. Technically, breakfast is important to have if it prevents overeating in the evening. Another reason to promote an earlier-eating window is that calories are burned more efficiently during the day than at night. Encourage your patients to take advantage of that. Calories are also burned more efficiently if they are consumed daily at the same time. This emphasizes the importance of having set mealtimes versus grazing. Grazing food throughout the day increases the risk of obesity by 57%.[13]

Not all studies show a positive benefit with intermittent fasting, and the studies that are promising are usually of short duration. Such is the case with most nutrition and exercise studies. This is why national guidelines and organizations may not fully endorse intermittent fasting. But that is a mistake. With possible benefits and minimal risks, if you can add this skill to your patients' repertoire, why not see if it can be helpful. Work with patients to see what they are willing to do and what can fit their lifestyle. Tell them that having an eating window of 10 hours (for example, 9 am to 7 pm) is the maximum recommended for benefits to begin and the earlier it is completed the better. Every patient will be different. Some get excited and go straight to a 6-hour eating window with no hesitation. Others will tread lightly and agree to a 10-hour window ending usually around 8 pm. Nudge them toward finishing a bit closer to 6 or 7 pm if you can. The first concern patients have when attempting time-restricted feeding is that they will get hungry. To your surprise, most people will not at all.

Not everyone can maintain a healthy eating window. With that in mind, one of the foremost longevity and fasting researchers Dr. Valter Longo introduced the world to the Fasting-Mimicking Diet (FMD). FMD in rodents reduced breast cancer and melanoma progression, increased life span, improved autoimmune diseases, reduced visceral fat and reversed type 1 and type 2 diabetes by regenerating beta cells in the pancreas.[14] In a study of 100 humans, FMD reduced body weight, BMI, body fat, IGF1 (Insulin like Growth Factor 1) and blood pressure but did not affect lipids, glucose or CRP.[15] Brandhorst et al. showed that three FMD cycles led to a 5.9% drop in fasting glucose, 15% reduction in IGF-1 levels (connected to cancer incidence), body weight reduced by 3% (mostly abdominal fat which is to be expected by a switch to a fatty acid catabolism mode) and CRP levels returned to normal in seven of eight patients with elevated baseline levels, and there were regenerative effects in humans due to seeing elevations in mesenchymal stem and progenitor cells (MSPC).

Based on the above, in addition to time-restricted feeding, ask your patients to try 5 days of a fasting-mimicking diet at least every 3 months. It is a nice way to reset the body and can be a starting point to get back on track for some patients.

How much to eat

There have been numerous studies looking at eating less calories and weight loss. On average it looks like there can be 5%–8% weight loss,[16] with a wide range of possible outcomes from 1% to 15%.[17] The exact deficit of calories needed depends on multiple factors including gender, age, current weight, muscle mass and weight goal. In general, most low-calorie diets involve 500–800 calories less than current caloric intake for the patient. Good numbers to keep in mind for our patients is 1,200–1,500 calories a day for women and 1,500–1,800 calories a day for men. Very low-calorie diets are defined as 800 calories a day or less. There are more extreme caloric restriction diets studied (500 calories a day) with great short-term weight loss success. Very low-calorie diets can be done as a jumpstart to success. How long to do it for is up to you and the patient. Anywhere from 5 days to 3 months is reasonable. Very low-calorie diets have shown no extra weight loss compared to low-calorie diets in the long term.[18] But success in that first month may be crucial.[19] That first month is when your patient has extra focus, and it would be prudent to take advantage of that while making it clear to the patient that sustainable changes are the real goal. A convenient way to have significantly less calories is meal replacements. Meal replacements have been clearly shown to help with weight loss. A meta-analysis showed that meal replacements with enhanced support led to 13 lbs more weight loss compared to other diets[20]—hence the many popular meal replacement commercial programs available to patients. The initial phase of weight loss with a very low-calorie diet can be all meal replacements. The advantage of medically supervised meal replacements is that it eliminates choices and is likely perfectly portioned (protein to carbohydrate ratio) with adequate micronutrients for good health outcomes while avoiding any complications. Strict meal replacement diets do require closer medical attention. That means vitals checks, monitoring blood pressure and blood glucose (glucose-lowering medications may need titration)·and checking basic labs such as CMP, magnesium and phosphorus on a weekly basis. Patients can be told that when they transition from a very low-calorie diet to a low-calorie diet (which is more sustainable), they can still do one or two meal replacements daily. Most patients welcome that idea as their day-to-day busy schedule can easily fit in a ready-to-eat or ready-to-drink supplement.

A common theme with most healthy lifestyle habits is that regardless of weight loss achieved, the habit itself leads to several good health outcomes. When you mention these other benefits to your patient, the hope is that one of them will trigger a strong motivation for change. Caloric restriction is no exception. Less calories daily can prolong your patient's life,[21] and this one possible benefit may be the impetus your patient needs to start having less calories. Kraus et al. in 2019 did the CALERIE study, where subjects had 25% less calories and results showed lower blood pressure, LDL cholesterol, total cholesterol to HDL ratio and improved insulin sensitivity.[22] Redman in 2011 indicated that risk of a heart attack or stroke can go down by as much as 30% after just 6 months of eating less calories.[23] That is a very vivid statement that can potentially hit home with your patients. Other potential benefits of having less calories include improved endothelial function,[24] lower muscle wasting with aging,[25] improved memory in the elderly, reduced systemic inflammation[26] and improved renal function.[27]

When discussing caloric restriction, it is a good time to highlight the importance of a well-rounded weight loss plan. Think about this. When it comes to lowering calories as part of a weight loss plan, there is not much selling you must do. Patients know they need to eat less. This is not a secret strategy that you are about to enlighten them with. Eating less has been a weight loss mantra since the 1940s and look where that has gotten society. The disease of obesity and environmental influences make the task of eating less very difficult in the short and long terms. In fact, adherence to an energy-restricted diet usually wanes in 1–4 months.[28] This must be clearly stated to your patient. What they are trying to do is hard. It is not their fault or their weakness that prevents them from sticking to the plan. This empathy is important. This act of normalizing their struggles is what will connect your patient to you and increase the likelihood of a successful partnership. It will also make clear to the patient that simply focusing on eating less and moving more may not be the best way forward. If you can achieve that breakthrough in their thought process, you may have unlocked their ability to succeed.

What to eat

This would be the billion-dollar question. Every year millions of people look for a specific diet that will help them lose weight. Whether it's a Ketogenic diet, Atkins, Paleo or Veganism. People become fixated with the specifics of a particular diet. Current evidence suggests that the best eating pattern for weight loss is the one the patient is willing to adhere too.[29] Not the answer you were looking for. Unfortunately, there is no one-size-fits-all way of losing weight. There have been numerous studies looking at macronutrient compositions (for example low fat vs low carbohydrate) and specific dietary patterns such as the Mediterranean diet, and there is no clear winner. In the short term (6 months or less), low carbohydrate seems to be better for weight loss,[30] but when looking at studies 1 year or longer, this advantage wanes.[31,32] So, what do you tell your patients? (Figure 4.1).

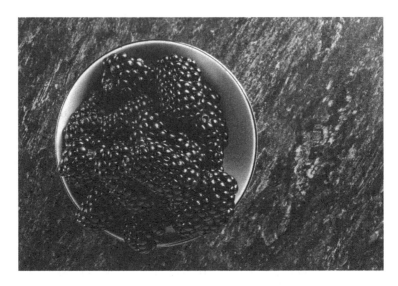

Figure 4.1 Berries, apples and pears are the fruits with a higher fiber content. Berries would be considered a super food based on the number of powerful antioxidant and anti-inflammatory molecules they contain. Ask your patients to include a cup of berries on most days of the week.

Patients can be educated on nutrition using macro- and micronutrient compositions (protein, fat, carbohydrate, water, fiber, vitamins, minerals, phytochemicals) or food groups (meat, poultry, fish, dairy, fruits, vegetables, legumes, whole grains, nuts, seeds, processed, ultraprocessed). Every physician or dietician has their own style and approach. There is technically no wrong or right way to discussing nutrition with your patient as the specific eating pattern does not seem to matter when it comes to weight loss. Lowering caloric intake, health-promoting foods, being physically active, improving sleep, reducing stress, behavioral therapy strategies and personalizing the plan would be factors that will make the best outcome possible for your patient. As such, it is a good idea to gauge what your patient is already thinking of, in terms of an eating plan, and what they have had success and failure with in the past. Remind them that regardless of what they have tried before, it is good to have an open mind. This will allow them to be in a better position to succeed this time. If the patient comes in with the idea of trying a low-carbohydrate diet or being vegetarian, then that is the starting point to work from. The next step is to focus on processed versus unprocessed foods.

Processed foods are any food item that has been altered from its natural, whole food state. There are degrees to the extent of processing, with ultraprocessed foods at an extreme end. To help the patient understand this important concept, a clear example can be useful. Take a whole apple. There is no ingredient list to this food item. Processing of this apple can then create (ordered from least processed to most processed) dried apples, apple sauce, natural apple juice, apple juice with added sugar, apple pie and then a hard apple candy. Your patient can now appreciate what a processed versus an unprocessed food would look like. Other examples of ultraprocessed foods include sweet or savory packaged snacks, sugar-sweetened beverages, candy, industrial bread, industrial breakfast cereal, ready-to-heat-and-eat pasta dishes and pizza, and sausages and other reconstituted meat products.[33] You want your patient to limit processed foods as best as they can. In a cohort study of over 44,000 French adults, a 10% increase in the proportion of ultraprocessed foods was associated with a 14% higher risk of all-cause mortality.[34] In a systematic review and meta-analysis of observational studies, there was a significant association between ultraprocessed foods and obesity.[35] Extra emphasis should be placed on avoiding or limiting processed meats (such as bacon, sausage, hot dogs and cold cuts). The World Health Organization has categorized processed meat as a Group 1 carcinogen due to its association with colon cancer.

A good way to help the patient reduce processed foods is to focus on the addition of healthy unprocessed foods. Now, it is easy to get lost in the idea of specific foods and how they may help with weight loss. For example, in a 2015 study by Hull et al., a handful of almonds in the morning led to less calories ingested at lunch and dinner due to increased satiety.[36] In a systematic review and meta-analysis in 2017, flaxseeds significantly improved weight loss, waist circumference and BMI versus lifestyle advice alone,[37] and in a 2009 study by Kondo et al., a tablespoon of vinegar daily was shown to lower weight and visceral fat by helping improve satiety.[38] But it is not necessary to focus on individual food items. It is also not necessary to focus on the macronutrient composition of the diet. Majority of patients will find it difficult to have a practical understanding of what a low-carbohydrate or low-fat or high-protein diet is. Maybe because there are no exact definitions. Low-carbohydrate diet can be less than 130 g a day, less than 50 g a day (for Atkins or keto-type diet usually) or less than 45% of the diet. Even the almost universally held belief that a high-protein diet (more than 25% of calories or about 70–100 g a day) is essential for weight loss is not based on concrete science.[39] Phone Apps have made it easier to monitor intake and see if your diet content is within these limits, but effort is required, nonetheless. Therefore, a shift has been made to focus on dietary patterns like the Mediterranean diet. Mancini et al. in 2016 did a systematic review of the Mediterranean diet and long-term weight loss.[40] It did help with weight loss (about 10–20 lbs) but not too different from other comparator diets. As such, even a popular dietary pattern has not stood out as head and shoulders above the rest.

Instead, why not take the foods common to various evidence-based diets (Mediterranean, DASH, Atkins, low glycemic, vegetarian, etc.) and make them the focus of a healthy calorie-reduced eating pattern. This would make the ideal dietary pattern plant-forward. This does not mean you have to eliminate animal-based products. That is an individual choice. But there is no doubt that drastically increasing certain fruits, vegetables, legumes, whole grains, nuts, seeds, herbs and spices will prove beneficial in a multitude of ways. You do still have to be calorie conscious. This is where the evidence-based volumetric diet started by Barbara Rolls at Penn State University can help inform us about the energy density of common foods.[41] For example, nuts and legumes (lentils, beans, chickpeas and split peas) should be a consistent part of a good eating pattern. A study showed that for every 20 g of legumes consumed, there was an 8% reduction in death.[42] Similarly, a study published in the *New England Journal of Medicine* in 2013 showed that nuts help lower mortality.[43] But during the weight loss phase, they need to be consumed in much smaller portions than commonly thought of.

Take advantage of the fiber, antioxidants and anti-inflammatory properties of plant-based foods as they likely help with weight loss in mechanisms that are yet to be discovered (Figure 4.2).

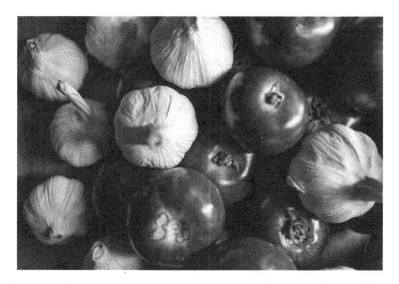

Figure 4.2 A nice way to start a weight loss eating plan is by asking patients to add healthy foods instead of asking them to stop eating unhealthy foods. When it comes to vegetables, think of the allium family (onion, garlic and leeks) as the one that offers the most antioxidant punch. But always ask them to have a variety of colors and see what vegetables they enjoy already based on their cultural foods.

Sedentary time

Sedentary time is the time your patient is sitting or lying down during awake hours. It has been formally defined as any waking behavior characterized by an energy expenditure ≤1.5 metabolic equivalents of task (METs) while in a seated, reclined or lying posture.[44] There has been a lot of emphasis on sedentary time recently. The new slogan of sitting is the new smoking, becoming a popular phrase. Think of sedentary time as a separate target and tool for obesity management in addition to aerobic and resistance training. There are two aspects to sedentary time: the total amount of sedentary time for the day, and the length of time for individual bouts of sitting. The goal is to reduce that total sedentary time to less than 8 hours and not sit for longer than 30 minutes at any time. In a meta-analysis by Biswas et al. in 2015, 14 studies on cardiovascular disease and diabetes, 14 studies on cancer and 13 studies on all-cause mortality were found.[45] There were significant associations found with all-cause mortality, cancer incidence and mortality, CV incidence and mortality and type 2 diabetes. Exercise did attenuate this risk but not completely. In another meta-analysis, 60–75 minutes of exercise negated the risk of more than 8 hours of sedentary time for all-cause mortality. But exercise did not negate the risk as well if the sedentary time involved watching TV. For those doing 60–75 minutes of activity, risk started to increase if there was 5 hours or more of TV watching time.[46] Both longer total sitting time and longer single bouts of sitting were deleteriously associated with fasting insulin, triglyceride, BMI, WC and insulin resistance.[47]

Reducing sedentary time is likely the first physical activity marker you and your patient can easily work on. Many of us have sedentary jobs, and in this new world of more people working from home, this has increased significantly. The key to improving this health parameter is to emphasize the importance of never sitting for longer than 30 minutes. This will be a bit perplexing to your patient. Thirty minutes is a very short amount of time. Office meetings, phone calls with friends or even a show on Netflix can last longer than 30 minutes. Tell your patient that even during those activities they must find a way to get up and move around. It will not be an easy habit to change. It will require constant reminders. A good trick is to write the words 'get up' on a post-it and have it on your desk or in the living room coffee table. Every time your patient sees it, they will be reminded that they must get up. The second strategy to help your patient improve sedentary time is to discuss adding more active leisure time activities. This will help reduce total sedentary time. This can be anything from scheduled exercise more often during the week to finally signing up for the ballroom dancing classes your patient has always wanted to do. This can be a fun part of the weight loss plan as your patient can explore activities they have never tried before and always wanted to do.

The final applicable strategy regarding sedentary time may be the most important. If you and your patient are struggling to reduce sedentary time, try to bargain with your patient and ask if they can give you 5–10 minutes of any type of activity after any meal or snack they consume. The patient can start with one specific meal such as dinner. But eventually at future office visits, you can add to this goal by asking the patient to be active after any calories they consume throughout the day. This is because the timing of this activity after meals may help with improving glycemic control and insulin resistance.[48] This may be an excellent strategy to keep in mind when dealing with patients who have diabetes and others who have subtle insulin resistance.

Aerobic activity

Aerobic activity is the usual form of activity recommended in combination with calorie restriction. On its own it can lead to a 6–7 lbs weight loss on average. In comparison, when aerobic activity is combined with caloric restriction, the average weight loss is closer to 20 lbs.[49] Thus, exercise is not the biggest weapon we have in combating weight loss. This is good information for your patients. It will be helpful to patients if they understand that nutrition is far more valuable to the weight loss plan. A lot of patients try to outrun their bad eating habits, and that mindset will only lead to a more difficult path to success. Aerobic activity, of course, has many benefits regardless of any effect on weight. For example, cardiorespiratory fitness (CRF) may be the best predictor of cardiovascular disease. Low CRF is also a risk factor for diabetes. Aerobic exercise improves CRF.[50] So aerobic exercise should never be discouraged even when a patient comes to you and says they have been active but have not seen any weight loss. These situations would be a good opportunity to discuss the other benefits of exercise, which are discussed in a bit more detail in the next chapter.

Your patient can be active in many ways such as walking, running, biking, hiking, swimming and elliptical use. The duration and intensity do matter. Exercise in bouts of 10 minutes minimum seems to have good benefits.[51] In fact, a large prospective study published in the *European Heart Journal* found that as little as 15 minutes/week of vigorous intensity activity was associated with a 16%–18% lower all-cause and cancer mortality.[52] Twenty minutes per week was associated with a 40% lower risk of cardiovascular death. That is a minuscule amount and very reasonable for patients. The total amount of aerobic activity recommended during the weight loss phase is about 150–300 minutes weekly.[53] The required amount of activity changes as your patient loses weight. In multiple studies, it has been seen that those who are successful in keeping the weight down are the ones who are most active. A good example of this is the subjects in the National Weight Control Registry. Individuals in this cohort have lost at least 30 lbs and kept it off for 5 years minimum. On average, the people in this group work out 60 minutes a day.[54] The recommended activity level during the weight maintenance phase is 300–420 minutes a week.[55] That is a considerable amount of activity, especially for people who have never been active. This is why discussing exercise early on can be beneficial in the long run. You want your patient to be in the habit of doing some exercise on a consistent basis by the time they have lost 10–20 lbs. This will allow them a better chance to reach that 300 minutes a week mark in hopes of retaining that weight loss.

The durations of aerobic exercise recommended so far are for moderate-intensity activity. This is subjective, but think of moderate intensity as an activity your patient can do while being a bit uncomfortable to talk. High-intensity activity, on the other hand, is activity that makes it very difficult to talk. If your patient prefers high-intensity workouts, then the recommended minutes per week are cut in half. This is one of the advantages of high-intensity interval training or HIIT. Less time investment is needed from your patient. If you have a patient who mentions on multiple office visits that they do not have time to exercise, introduce them to HIIT. Let them know they can get equal benefits in half the time. A meta-analysis showed that HIIT provided similar benefits to moderate-intensity aerobic exercise for improving body composition, VO2max and total cholesterol.[56] That may be the information they need to start being more active.

The best aerobic activity your patient can do is the one they are willing to do. Enjoyment level matters as that indicates sustainability of that activity. And there is a dose–response relationship so that the more activity your patient does, the higher the weight loss potential.[57] Make aerobic activity essential to your plan.

Resistance training

This includes bodyweight training, isometric exercises (such as with bands) and weight training. The evidence that resistance training alone can help with weight loss is poor.[58] When added to aerobic training or caloric restriction, there is very little additional benefit in terms of weight loss according to several RCTs.[59,60] But this is the issue with having weight as the only parameter of concern. The focus on weight ignores all the other benefits of resistance training which would be a shame to ignore for our patients. In a meta-analysis,

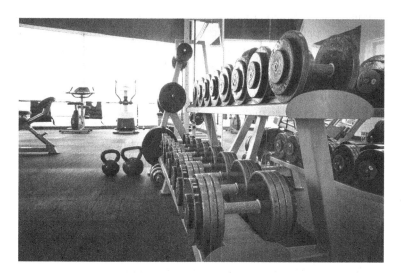

Figure 4.3 Any amount of activity is helpful for the overall health of your patient. Numerous studies have now confirmed that even a little bit of activity can go a long way to reducing mortality. But for weight loss, exercise is not considered a major weapon. Do not let that stop you from bringing up exercise and reducing sedentary time with your patient.

muscle-strengthening activities were associated with a 15% lower risk of all-cause mortality.[61] Excess adipose tissue is what obesity is, and specifically, excess adipose tissue in the abdomen is associated with worse health outcomes. Resistance training has been shown to reduce body fat and visceral adipose tissue.[62] We know sleep is connected to obesity, and sleep quality and duration are both improved with resistance training.[63,64] Depression and anxiety, when present, hinder progress with more episodes of emotional eating and lack of compliance with healthy lifestyle habits. In a meta-analysis, both depression[65] and anxiety[66] improve with resistance training. One of the main reasons we care about weight loss for our patients is to improve cardiometabolic parameters. Resistance training works just as well as aerobic exercise for NAFLD, and maybe even better because it requires less intensity.[67] It reduces risk of diabetes and cardiovascular disease independent of aerobic activity.[68] Both resistance and aerobic exercise work equally as well for glycemic control and lipid parameters.[69] Both resistance and aerobic exercise can lower blood pressure almost as much as blood pressure medications.[70] Maybe the benefit that can be emphasized the most with your patient is improved cardiorespiratory fitness, which is independent of aerobic activity.[71] As we learned above that cardiorespiratory fitness is clearly connected to all-cause mortality.[72] Use the above benefits of resistance training to motivate your patient to incorporate this as part of their weight loss plan. The improvement in self-efficacy alone may be worth it (Figure 4.3).[73]

Resistance training can be daunting for patients who have never done it before. Encourage your patient to find a friend or family member who has experience and to work out with them initially. They can also get a personal trainer in the beginning to learn proper form and techniques to prevent injury. The minimum sessions a week ideally is 2–3. The duration of each session is whatever the patient is willing to do, but minimum to be encouraged is 10 minutes. Let the patient know they can do resistance training on consecutive days if they are working on different parts of the body such as upper body one day and the next day is lower body. This allows for proper muscle recovery. Thus, a workout regimen with 150–300 minutes of moderate-intensity aerobic activity in combination with 2–3 days of resistance training for minimum of 10 minutes would be excellent to promote to our patients.

Sleep

You can live without food for weeks and without water for days, but try not to sleep at all and your experimentation (and life!) may come to a halt very soon. It is crazy to think how much we ignore and de-prioritize an aspect of life that takes up one-third of our entire time on earth. Sleep should be one of the pillars you lean on when it comes to weight loss for your patients (Figure 4.4).

You can tell patients that the ideal amount of sleep for weight loss is around 7.5–9 hours.[74] Just one night of poor sleep leads to increased cravings for fatty and sugar-dense foods[75,76] and wanting larger portions of food.[77] This is essential information for your patient. It will allow them to be more aware of how they eat the day after a disturbed night of sleep. Poor sleep also leads to less fat burning during sleep, and more muscle mass loss.[78,79,80] Now imagine weeks to months to years of inadequate sleep and how that would impact a person's ability to stick to their weight loss–related behavior goals. The underlying mechanisms on why bad sleep

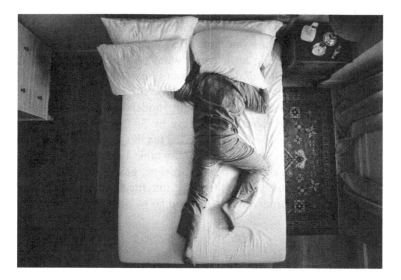

Figure 4.4 Make it a point to let your patient know early on that quality sleep and reducing stress are as important to the weight loss effort as reducing calories and exercising more. If you can do this, success for your patient will be much more likely.

can worsen eating behavior include findings that sleeping close to 6 hours or less leads to a 15% increase in ghrelin (the hunger hormone) and a similar decrease in leptin (the satiety hormone). Explain this physiology to your patient.

Now, if you notice your patient not really paying attention to the sleep and obesity paradigm, then a good way to engage the patient is connecting poor sleep to something that matters to them. Specific reasons you can mention to your patient on why sleep is important include insufficient sleep leads to increased mortality,[81] risk for Alzheimer's disease,[82] acute cognitive decline and attention deficit,[83] higher suicide risk,[84,85] depression,[86] anxiety,[87] higher heart rate and blood pressure,[88] more coronary artery calcification,[89] more heart attacks,[90] immune system suffers and diseases like COVID-19 can be more of a concern, insulin resistance worsens,[91] testosterone levels decrease in men to those of people 10 years older,[92] sperm quality and quantity decrease,[93] menstrual irregularities,[94] worsened reaction times and visual attention and hence more car accidents,[95] and being less attractive.[96]

For counseling patients on good sleep habits, some key concepts include taking advantage of the circadian rhythm (going to bed and waking up at the same time regardless of weekday, weekend, vacation, etc.), having an evening wind down routine (dimming lights, no exercise/food/alcohol 3 hours before bedtime), reducing all sensory stimulation (quiet and dark room, comfortable bed, turning all electronics into red light mode), temperature regulation (lowering the room temperature by 3–4 degrees 30 minutes before bedtime, hot bath, warm herbal tea like chamomile, less salt and carbohydrates for dinner, comfortable blankets) and reducing stress (no work emails before bedtime, gratitude journal right before bed, progressive muscle relaxation, meditation and avoiding ruminating/planning/worrying as you go to bed).

Stress

This may be the most difficult aspect of obesity management to grasp but the most important one to master. It is easy to understand how eating less and moving more may be connected to weight loss. Despite this obvious relationship, most individuals struggle to lose weight. One of the many reasons is stress, more specifically chronic mental stress. Stress activates the hypothalamic-pituitary-adrenal axis with the end products of cortisol and norepinephrine causing chaos. This is a multi-pronged attack on the body that leads to perpetual obesity. The elevated levels of cortisol and norepinephrine lead to poor executive function (ability to make healthy lifestyle choices compromised),[97] hunger for foods rich in fat and added sugars (making it harder to stick to a healthy food plan),[98,99] any underlying anxiety/depression worsens (again, making it more difficult to want to stay on a healthy lifestyle plan), white adipose tissue in the body gets redistributed to visceral abdominal fat (making it more likely to have the comorbid conditions of metabolic syndrome and heart disease)[100] and affects sleep duration and quality (which we have learned in the previous section as an integral component for weight loss success).[101] What makes this even more difficult is that a vicious cycle ensues whereby the obesity itself (due to inner negative self-talk, poor body image, poor self-efficacy, and the daily struggles of weight stigmata) leads to more stress. Hence, the ill effect of cortisol is sustained.

As you try to appreciate the difficult position your patient is in when it comes to stress and trying to lose weight, let's add other layers of complexity. Stress is universal, subjective, difficult to measure, and hard to explain to your patient. With the information in this chapter, you may now be able to help your patient understand in simple terms that there is a connection between stress and obesity. But then comes the final hurdle. Your patient will say 'Doc, my job is stressful,' 'I'm in a difficult relationship,' or 'I am studying for exams and stressed out.' What do you say now?

This is what makes obesity management hard. You know that reducing stress can help your patient lose weight. You may even have convinced the patient the importance of stress management in their weight loss journey. But life circumstances won't allow the stressors to go away, and even if a specific stressor does go away or improve, another stressor will pop up in its place in due time. You must explain this never-ending nature of stress to the patient. Once you do, you tell them that this is what makes losing weight and maintaining a good weight such a difficult task. But success will be more likely if we can incorporate stress-reducing activities into their daily routine.

All the lifestyle habits are intertwined, and so by improving nutrition, activity levels and sleep, stress naturally will go down. The next two biggest tools to help reduce stress are mindfulness and meditation. Think of mindfulness as the act of really paying attention to any action that you are doing without any judgment. Mindfulness can help improve sleep,[102] lower cortisol levels and improve cognitive function.[103] All things that aid in obesity management and so there is no surprise that mindfulness has been shown to help with weight loss.[104] There are self-help books your patient can use to learn mindfulness, or you can connect them with a mindfulness expert locally. Meditation is basically a form of mindfulness. There are excellent commercial apps that help with this practice such as Calm and Headspace. You can ask your patient to do 3 minutes before bedtime daily as a starting point. In a meta-analysis and systematic review by Goyal et al. in 2014, meditation was found to have a small to moderate effect on psychological stress.[105] There are different forms of meditation, and mindfulness meditation specifically has been connected to improvement in emotional eating and binge eating in a systematic review done by Katterman et al. in 2014.[106] In that study, the results were mixed when looking at weight loss alone. Other stress-reducing activities to encourage for your patients can include yoga, tai chi, massage therapy, floatation therapy, art therapy, music therapy, acts of kindness,[107] spending time with friends/family,[108] gratitude journal,[109] volunteering, time in nature and valuing time over money.[110]

Obesity pharmacotherapy

Think of anti-obesity medications like you would for any other chronic disease. If you diagnose someone with primary hypertension and their blood pressure is consistently over 160/100, you will not hesitate to start medications. If blood pressure is mildly elevated, you may ask your patient to try to improve their lifestyle habits for 3–6 months, and if no improvement, then medications will be started. If after adding a blood pressure medication, the blood pressure is still not controlled, you add a second medication, while you continue to encourage healthy habits. Your thought process can be the same when treating obesity.

At a BMI of 30 and above, your patient qualifies for weight loss medications. If the BMI is above 27, then another comorbid condition is required. Only 1% of people who qualify for an obesity medication are currently getting them right now.[111] We have much to improve on. You can be a part of the solution.

Once started on a weight loss medication, success is considered when 5% weight loss is achieved in 3 months. If this is not achieved, then discontinuing medication should be discussed. It is important to note that no weight loss medication is safe during pregnancy.

We are in the nascent stages of obesity pharmacology as we slowly understand the disease process, and breakthrough therapeutic targets are coming into action. Be prepared for a new horizon over the next decade.

FDA-approved medication

Adipex (Phentermine)

Mechanism of Action – Inhibits dopamine and serotonin reuptake and is weakly adrenergic.

Dosing – Start with 15 mg once daily in the morning. Effects last about 12 hours so can impact sleep if taken later in the day. If 5% weight loss achieved, this is a good dose to stay at long term and no need to increase to the higher dose of 30 or 37.5 mg. There is a brand version of phentermine called Lomaira that is an 8 mg tablet and can be taken up to three times a day.

Things to know – This is a controlled substance, and most states require prescriptions be for 30 days with no refills. If using longer than 3 months, which is very likely, document that it is off-label use in chart. Not ideal for patients who drink a lot of caffeine, have uncontrolled high blood pressure, or have anxiety, insomnia, hyperthyroidism, glaucoma or coronary artery disease. Ideal for young and healthy patients, especially if there is low energy and motivation. Average weight loss in a review of RCTs was 0.6–6 kg.[112] A caveat to keep in mind is that intermittent use, such as weekends only, can be effective for some patients.[113]

Xenical or Alli (Orlistat)

Mechanism of Action – Pancreatic lipase inhibitor. Blocks absorption of about 30% of dietary fat.

Dosing – 60 mg TID from OTC is called Alli, and prescription dose is called Xenical 120 mg TID.

Things to know – Prescribed less frequently due to common side effects of flatulence, diarrhea, bloating and abdominal cramping. If prescribed, make sure to also prescribe multivitamins to be taken at least 2 hours after orlistat intake, to prevent deficiency of fat-soluble vitamins. Can be beneficial for patients with hypertriglyceridemia. Average weight loss of 2.6 kg after 1 year.[114]

Contrave (Naltrexone/Bupropion)

Mechanism of Action – A combination drug of naltrexone 8 mg and bupropion 90 mg. Bupropion is the main ingredient as it directly activates a part of the brain that reduces hunger and increases energy expenditure. The naltrexone helps by prolonging the effect of bupropion in the brain. The naltrexone itself can be beneficial for weight loss, but its exact mechanism is unknown.

Dosing – 1 tablet in the morning in week 1, then twice a day in week 2, then 2 tablets in the morning and one in the evening in week 3, and finally 2 tablets twice a day thereafter. In patients with renal or liver dysfunction, 1 tablet BID recommended maintenance dose.

Things to know – Remember to avoid this medication in anyone taking opioids for long term. Remind patients that if acute pain issues arise such as a fracture, opioids will be less effective due to the naltrexone. Not ideal for patients with insomnia, high blood pressure, seizure history, bulimia and anxiety. But this would be ideal for those trying to quit smoking, needing to lower alcohol intake, having depression and those with excessive cravings. Average weight loss of 5 kg after 1 year.[115] Another way to educate patients on the effectiveness of this medication can be that 50% of people lose at least 5% of their weight.[116]

Qsymia (Phentermine/Topiramate)

Mechanism of action – Please see mechanism of action of the individual components.

Dosing – Take one 3.75 mg/23 mg capsule daily for 2 weeks and then increase dose to 7.5 mg/46 mg daily thereafter. If less than 5% weight loss over 3 months, then can change dose to 11.25 mg/69 mg for 2 weeks and then increase again to the maximum dose of 15mg/92 mg thereafter.

Things to know – Most people do well on the 7.5 mg/46 mg once daily dose for the long term. After semaglutide 2.4 mg (Wegovy), this medication is the most effective for weight loss (about 12% weight loss). In a meta-analysis, it was shown to have 8.8 kg of weight loss on average after a year.[117]

Saxenda (Liraglutide)

Mechanism of action – Glucagon-like peptide (GLP)-1 receptor agonist. Directly suppresses appetite and boosts energy metabolism by going to the hypothalamus, slows gastric emptying during meals, reduces gluconeogenesis in the liver and turns up insulin production to just the right amount needed for metabolism after food consumption.

Dosing – You may be familiar with Victoza for patients with diabetes. That is liraglutide that goes to a maximum dose of 1.8 mg. Saxenda goes to 3 mg as its maximum dose. Titration starts at 0.6 mg once daily subcutaneous injection in outer thigh, abdomen or triceps area for 7 days, then 1.2 mg daily for 7 days, then 1.8 mg daily for 7 days, then 2.4 mg daily for 7 days and then finally the highest dose of 3 mg daily thereafter.

Things to know – Common side effects to look for in all GLP1 agonists are nausea and constipation. Not ideal for patients with history of pancreatitis, gastroparesis or severe heartburn. GLP1 agonists are contraindicated in patients with a family or personal history of medullary thyroid cancer or multiple endocrine neoplasia. The original RCT was called SCALE, and in this 56 week study, the average weight loss was 8.4 kg. A total of 63.2% patients lost at least 5% of their original weight, while 33.1% of patients lost at least 10% of their weight.[118] These are the weight loss estimates you can tell your patients.

Wegovy (Semaglutide)

Mechanism of action – Please see the mechanism of action for Saxenda.

Dosing – Subcutaneous injection of 0.25 mg once weekly in outer thigh, abdomen or triceps for 4 weeks, then 0.5 mg once weekly for 4 weeks, then 1 mg once weekly for 4 weeks, then 1.7 mg once weekly for 4 weeks and then finally the highest dose of 2.4 mg weekly thereafter. If patient is successful at a lower dose such as 1 or 1.7 mg, then it is more than appropriate to stay at that dose and not titrate like clockwork all the way up to 2.4 mg.

Things to know – Fifty percent of patients lose at least 15% with one-third of patients losing more than 20%.[119] The average weight loss was 15.3 kg at 68 weeks in the STEP 1 trial. Our best tool yet, in terms of ease of use, efficacy and side-effect profile.

Vyvanse (Lisdexamfetamine)

Mechanism of action – A central nervous system stimulant that causes appetite suppression.

Dosing – Start at 30 mg once daily. Can be titrated weekly by 10–20 mg to a target dose of 50–70 mg once daily.

Things to know – FDA approved for Binge-Eating Disorder and not for obesity. Studies have shown it helps lower the frequency of binge-eating episodes.[120] Ideal for patients who mention attention-deficit disorder symptoms. Not ideal for those with anxiety, insomnia or high blood pressure.

Off-label medications

Metformin

Mechanism of action – For weight loss, it is unknown but likely related to lowering insulin resistance through decreased glucose production by the liver, increased glucose uptake by the muscle and blocking glucose absorption in the intestines.

Dosing – We are all familiar with metformin. The dose that can possibly curb appetite is 1,500 mg daily.[121] Extended release preferred to prevent side effects.

Things to know – To reduce gastrointestinal side effects early on, advise your patient to take with food only and lower overall carbohydrate intake. Add vitamin B12 supplementation as metformin can reduce absorption of vitamin B12. Avoid if GFR less than 30. The studies on metformin and weight loss are mixed. Anywhere from weight neutral[122] to 3.8 kg of weight loss.[123] A good opportunity to use metformin is in patients taking atypical anti-psychotics. In a meta-analysis, metformin was shown to reduce BMI and insulin resistance in patients on atypical anti-psychotics.[124]

Other GLPI agonists like Victoza, Trulicity, etc.

All GLP1 agonists have the potential for helping with weight loss. See Saxenda (Liraglutide) for details.

SGLT2 inhibitors

Mechanism of action – It prevents reabsorption of filtered glucose in the kidney. Weight loss mechanism is unknown but likely related to lowering insulin resistance. The average weight loss measured for dapagliflozin and canagliflozin stands between 1% and 3%, while other reports mention a loss greater than 5%.[125]

Topiramate

Mechanism of action – Unknown mechanism of action. Helps reduce hunger and cravings.

Dosing – Start at 25 mg once daily but can be titrated to 200 mg a day in two divided doses. Majority of patients can do well on 25 mg once a day only or 25–50 mg BID. Usually, no need to go higher than that.

Things to know – Avoid in patients with history of kidney stones. If this medication needs to be stopped, taper off slowly due to risk of seizures with abrupt withdrawals. Main side effects to mention to the patient include drowsiness, paresthesia (tingling in the hands and feet) and slowing of cognition.

Zonisamide

Mechanism of action – It enhances serotonin and dopamine activities in the brain.

Dosing – Start at 25 mg once daily, and most patients do well with 100 mg or less. Maximum dose of 400 mg.

Things to know – Zonisamide is similar to topiramate in action and side effects. Both can help with sleep if taken in evening.

Bupropion

Mechanism of action – Dopamine and norepinephrine reuptake inhibitor. It also stimulates POMC in the hypothalamus and leads to less hunger and increased resting metabolic rate.

Dosing – Start at 150 mg daily. Maximum dose of 450 mg daily.

Things to know – Useful if patient has co-morbidities of depression or tobacco use. Not recommended in patients with history of seizures or bulimia. Not ideal for patients with severe anxiety or insomnia.

Naltrexone

Mechanism of action – Unknown mechanism but likely to decrease the pleasure of excess foods.

Dosing – Start at 25 mg daily orally for one week and then increase to 50 mg daily thereafter.

Things to know – Avoid opioids during use. No significant side effects. This medication is more commonly used to help patients reduce alcohol intake. If your patient is currently using alcohol and they are in the mindset of slowing their intake, this would be an excellent choice. Also a good option if excess cravings are mentioned by your patient.

Combination therapy

Many of the FDA-approved medications are already a combination of medications. Qsymia is a combination of phentermine and topiramate. Contrave is a combination of bupropion and naltrexone. With a disease as complex as obesity, it makes sense that multiple mechanisms of action are at play. As a result, using multiple medications would be a good thought. Almost all the anti-obesity medications can be used together in various combinations. Start with a single medication, and if the minimum of 5% weight loss is reached, but the patient has not reached their goal weight, this would be an opportunity to add a second medication. Think of bupropion and phentermine as stimulant medications, and their use together would not be ideal as it may worsen any underlying anxiety and increase heart rate or blood pressure. Polypharmacy is always on our radar, but if the benefits outweigh the risks, do not hesitate. As your patient loses more weight and maintains that weight loss for a significant amount of time, a weight loss medication can be stopped if the lifestyle habits have noticeably changed. But let the patient know that there is no cure for obesity and long-term use is recommended and safe.

The future

The future is bright. We only have a handful of FDA-approved weight loss medications at the moment, but there are ongoing trials of some very promising medications.

Tirzepatide is a dual GLP1/GIP agonist. It is currently being studied to help with Hgb A1c (SURPASS clinical trials), weight loss (SURMOUNT clinical trials) and fatty liver (SYNERGY-NASH trial). Current dosing regimens include a starting dose of 2.5 mg subq injection weekly that is increased by 2.5 mg every 4 weeks to maintenance doses of 5, 10 or 15 mg. In a phase 2 trial, it was seen that the 15 mg dose led to an average weight loss of 11.3 kg.[126] In the SURPASS 2 trial, a phase 3 trial, 5, 10 or 15 mg of tirzepatide was compared to 1 mg of semaglutide.[127] Mean weight loss was higher in all tirzepatide groups with 11.2 kg seen in the 15 mg group.

Canagliflozin 300 mg plus phentermine 15 mg is a combination drug. Mean body weight change of 7.5% came to 7.3 kg at 26 weeks. One-third of patients lost at least 10% of body weight.[128] This amount of weight loss indicates an additive effect of the two medications.

Cagrilintide plus semaglutide 2.4 mg. Cagrilintide is a long-acting amylin. On its own, it has been shown to help with weight loss, with the 4.5 mg once weekly dose showing better efficacy than liraglutide 3 mg.[129] Six different doses of cagrilintide were studied in combination with semaglutide 2.4 mg. The 1.2 and 2.4 mg doses of cagrilintide once weekly in combination with semaglutide 2.4 mg once weekly showed a 15.7% and 17.1% average weight loss at 20 weeks, respectively.[130] This level of consistent weight loss would be exciting news.

Other anti-obesity drugs in the pipeline include centrally acting agents (setmelanotide, neuropeptide Y antagonist, zonisamide-bupropion, cannabinoid type-1 receptor blockers), amylin mimetics (davalintide, dual amylin and calcitonin receptor agonists), dual-action GLP-1/glucagon receptor agonists (oxyntomodulin) and other novel targets including anti-obesity vaccines (ghrelin, somatostatin, adenovirus36). With these new drugs in development, anti-obesity therapeutics have the potential for a more personalized approach to obesity care.[131]

Bariatric surgery

You may come across patients in your practice who have a history of bariatric surgery. Patients may also walk into your clinic curious about what surgery options they have for weight loss. Understanding some of the basics of bariatric surgery is important to help these patients. A lot of these patients with bariatric surgery have not seen their surgeon in a while for numerous reasons. You can offer them proper follow-up care as you help them establish again with a local bariatric surgeon (Figure 4.5).

Patients qualify for bariatric surgery if their BMI is over 40 or BMI over 35 with a comorbid condition. Common comorbid conditions that usually are accepted include hypertension, hyperlipidemia, diabetes and obstructive sleep apnea. In addition to the BMI qualifier, patients must be competent enough to understand the risks and benefits of surgery, have attempted medical weight loss for 6 months at least, have no recent suicide attempt or mental health hospitalization and no active substance abuse.

The two main surgeries to remember are sleeve gastrectomy (61% of all bariatric surgeries) and gastric bypass (17% of all bariatric surgeries; with another 15% of all bariatric surgeries being revisions). It is easier to understand these surgeries while looking at a picture. The sleeve gastrectomy is basically where the stomach is cut into the shape of a medium-sized banana. As

TYPES OF BARIATRIC SURGERY

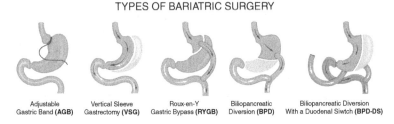

| Adjustable Gastric Band (AGB) | Vertical Sleeve Gastrectomy (VSG) | Roux-en-Y Gastric Bypass (RYGB) | Biliopancreatic Diversion (BPD) | Biliopancreatic Diversion With a Duodenal Siwtch (BPD-DS) |

Figure 4.5 A simple illustration of the available bariatric surgeries.

such, the overall anatomy of the digestive system remains intact. The area that is cut out had cells that released the hormone ghrelin (the hunger hormone). The ghrelin hormone rises slowly after meals and peaks right before the next meal as it makes you hungry. Without ghrelin, some patients after sleeve gastrectomy must be reminded to eat at consistent times with an alarm clock. So, this procedure helps with weight loss by being restrictive (smaller stomach), and there is a metabolic aspect to it. The surgery takes about an hour, you stay in the hospital overnight and full recovery can be expected in 3 weeks.

The gastric bypass procedure is more invasive. In this surgery, most of the stomach and duodenum are bypassed. To visualize this, think of the first step as cutting completely near the top of the stomach so that it is completely separated from the esophagus. Now think of the next step as the small intestine is cut completely in half soon after the jejunum begins. You now have floating around and attached to nothing, the entire stomach and duodenum. To make this whole again, the bottom portion of the cut small intestine is brought all the way up to attach to the esophagus. Now the duodenum part of the small intestine is important as that is where pancreatic juices enter the gut. They will be needed for digestion. So that part of the small intestine is attached again to the small intestine but much further down, closer to the large intestine. If you are wondering, much of the stomach that is attached to the duodenum remains floating in the body. Even though it is more invasive, due to improvements in technique and modern technology, most patients stay overnight only or 2–3 days maximum, and recovery is about 4–6 weeks for this procedure which takes about 2 hours in the operating room.

Patients lose on average 25%–30% of pre-operative weight with both these surgeries. The most common reasons for insufficient weight loss are no exercise and snacking.[132] Randomized trials comparing sleeve gastrectomy and gastric bypass show similar weight loss, while observational studies show that gastric bypass patients achieve greater weight loss than sleeve gastrectomy patients.[133] The benefits of this weight loss include remission of many medical problems, increased self-efficacy and helping the patient live longer. The Swedish Obesity Study showed a 29% reduction in death,[134] while Adams et al. in a retrospective study of 7,900 patients found a 40% reduction in mortality.[135] There have been 12 RCTs comparing surgical to medical treatment of type 2 diabetes. All but one showed surgery was superior. On average, surgery decreased A1c by 1.8%–3.5%, while medical treatments on average improve Hgb A1c by 0.4%–1.5%. This improvement in glycemic control is similar for both types of surgeries, but longer remission is seen with gastric bypass.[136] When it comes to dyslipidemia, a recent meta-analysis of RCTs comparing gastric bypass to sleeve gastrectomy found that resolution of dyslipidemia was higher with gastric bypass at 1 and 5 years,[137] but a different meta-analysis that included observational studies found no significant difference between the two surgeries at 3 years.[138] Systematic reviews indicate that 1-year hypertension remission rates range from 43% to 83% with the higher rates more likely with gastric bypass than sleeve gastrectomy.[139] Finally, obesity is associated with increased risk for several types of cancers. Data from eight observational studies suggest that bariatric surgery is associated with reduced risk of all types of cancers.[140]

The above benefits must be weighed against the potential risks. Overall, the literature supports that short- and long-term complications are greater with gastric bypass than sleeve gastrectomy.[141] The one advantage of gastric bypass is in the risk of weight regain back to the original pre-operative weight. This occurs in 3.3% of gastric bypass patients and 12.5% of sleeve gastrectomy patients.[142] The peri-operative (within 30 days of the operation) complications that can occur with both procedures include death (0.03%–0.2%), leaks (1%–2%), wound infections (1%–2%), DVT/PE (1%–2%) and nausea/vomiting/dehydration (1%–2%). The types of long-term complications differ between the two surgeries. The sleeve has minimal risks such as stenosis

(1%–2%), but the one common long-term risk to keep in mind is worsening GERD. This is a reason why patients with severe GERD may prefer gastric bypass over sleeve gastrectomy. As for the long-term complications for gastric bypass, they can include ulcers (3%–5%), small bowel obstructions (1%), internal hernias (1%–2%), incisional hernias (0.8%), stenosis/strictures (2%) and vitamin/nutrient deficiencies (15%–40%).

Other

A biliopancreatic diversion (BPD) is a third form of bariatric surgery but comprises less than 1% of all bariatric surgeries. You may also see patients with a history of a lap band procedure (2%–3% of all bariatric procedures). Lap bands used to be the most popular weight loss procedure and now has fallen out of favor due to high complication and reoperation rates.

Post-operative management

If you come across a patient within 1 year of their bariatric surgery, ask them if they are regularly following up with their surgeon. Ideally, bariatric surgeons are supposed to follow their patient for 5 years post op. The initial visits are at 1 week, 6 weeks, 3 months, 6 months, 9 months and 1 year. After that, yearly visits are adequate. Labs are ordered every 3 months within the first year and then yearly after that. Routine labs after bariatric surgery include CBC, CMP, lipid panel, Hgb A1c, iron studies, ferritin, vitamin D-25, vitamin B12, RBC-folate, thiamine, vitamin A, copper, magnesium, phosphorus, zinc, calcium, albumin, prealbumin and intact PTH. These are the labs to order during the annual visit if you have a patient who has a history of gastric bypass surgery. After a sleeve gastrectomy, the rarer mineral deficiencies, such as copper and zinc, do not have to be investigated for unless there is anemia without a confirmed cause. To help prevent these deficiencies altogether, dietary supplementation is important. All bariatric surgery patients need to take the following supplements for the rest of their life: 2 daily multivitamins with or without iron, 1,000–2,000 mg of calcium citrate, and vitamin D 3,000 units daily; supplementation can also be taken for vitamin B12 1,000 mcg IM monthly or 500 μg orally daily, folic acid 400 μg to 1 mg and a B complex.

CASE STUDY CONTINUED

In our visit with Martha, our lovely patient, we have so far discussed our medical assessment, made an initial treatment goal and explained the disease of obesity in simple terms. Next, we discuss treatment options.

Dr. C: To help with weight loss, we must think of three strategies. Lifestyle habits, anti-obesity medications and weight loss surgery. Based on your clinical history, you would qualify for weight loss surgery. There are two main types of surgery. One is called sleeve gastrectomy, and the other is called gastric bypass surgery. Think of the sleeve as making the stomach the size of a banana. By doing this, it restricts the amount of food you can have that makes you full. Also, the part of the stomach removed used to make a hormone that would make you hungry (Ghrelin). Without that hormone being released, the hunger levels go down. As for the gastric bypass, it is a more invasive procedure and works by restricting the food intake and by changing the hormones in the body. We can discuss that in more detail if you would like. Would surgery for weight loss be of interest to you?

M: No. I would like to avoid surgery, if possible.

Dr. C: No problem. Moving on to medications. There are five FDA-approved weight loss medications. I am going to say a bunch of names now. Stay with me. Orlistat, Contrave, Qsymia, Wegovy and Saxenda. There is also another medication that can work short and long terms, called phentermine. They all work in slightly different ways and come with different risks and side effects, which we can discuss in detail. Are you interested in medications for weight loss?

M: I definitely am. I have heard of phentermine. Also, a friend of mine is on Wegovy and has had lots of success. So I would be interested in learning about that.

Dr. C: Ok, I am glad you mentioned Wegovy or Semaglutide. That is the one I would recommend first for you. This is because you have prediabetes. Which tells me insulin resistance is hindering your ability to lose weight. And we need to counteract that. This medication will help in this regard. It works by slowing the stomach down so that food you eat sits there longer and makes you full. It also goes to the part of the brain that makes you less hungry. And finally, it helps reverse insulin resistance. It is a once weekly injection that you inject in the outer thigh or abdomen.

M: Sounds good to me. What are the side effects?

Dr. C: Good question. The most common side effects are nausea and constipation. But we slowly increase the dose to help minimize that. One thing we do have to mention is that there is a rare chance of a thyroid tumor called medullary thyroid cancer. But I have to say in the decades-long existence of this type of medication, it has not resulted in a single case in humans. It was found in rats on initial testing, and so we need to mention it.

M: Fair enough. I would like to start it. How much weight can I expect to lose?

Dr. C: On average, 15% of weight loss is expected, and in one-third of patients, the weight loss can be over 20%.

M: How long do I have to stay on the medication?

Dr. C: Another good question. Different doctors may think of this in different ways. There is technically no cure for obesity. So if the medication works, you can stay on it long term, just as you would a blood pressure or cholesterol medication. But if you had the desire to go off it, you can. I always tell patients that if you have successfully lost weight that you are happy with and kept it off for 6 to 12 months, then we can go off the medication.

M: I hope my insurance covers it.

Dr. C: I hope so too. I will go ahead and prescribe it now. Let's follow up in 2–4 weeks.

M: Appreciate your time and thorough explanations Dr. Chatterjee. I feel good about this.

Dr. C: My pleasure. Please take care.

NOTES

1 Rueda-Clausen et al. *Clinical Obesity* (2014). PMID: 25425131
2 Loprinzi et al. *American Journal of Health Promotion* (2016). DOI: 10.1177/0890117116646340
3 Rynders et al. *Nutrients* (2019). PMID: 31614992

4 Moro et al. *Journal of Translational Medicine* (2016). PMID: 27737674

5 Cienfuegos et al. *Cell Metabolism* (2020). PMID: 32673591

6 Li et al. *Cell Metabolism* (2017). PMID: 28918936

7 Sutton et al. *Cell Metabolism* (2018). PMID: 29754952

8 Gill et al. *Cell Metabolism* (2015). PMID: 26411343

9 Longo et al. *Cell Metabolism* (2016). PMID: 27304506

10 Ravussin et al. *Obesity* (2019). PMID: 31339000

11 Sutton et al. *Cell Metabolism* (2018). PMID: 29754952

12 Jones et al. *The American Journal of Clinical Nutrition* (2020). PMID: 32729615

13 Leech et al. *The American Journal of Clinical Nutrition* (2017). PMID: 28814392

14 Brandhorst et al. *Cell Metabolism* (2015). PMID: 26094889

15 Wei et al. *Science Translational Medicine* (2017). PMID: 28202779

16 Varady. *Obesity Reviews* (2011). PMID: 21410865

17 Zubrzycki et al. *Journal of Physiology and Pharmacology* (2018). PMID: 30683819

18 Freire. *Nutrition* (2020). PMID: 31525701

19 Unick et al. *Obesity* (2014). PMID: 24771618

20 Astbury et al. *Obesity Reviews* (2019). PMID: 30675990

21 Weindruch et al. *The New England Journal of Medicine* (1997). PMID: 9309105

22 Kraus et al. *The Lancet: Diabetes and Endocrinology* (2019). PMID: 31303390

23 Redman et al. *Antioxidants and Redox Signaling* (2011). PMID: 20518700

24 Garcia-Prieto et al. *Vascular Pharmacology* (2015). PMID: 25530153

25 McKiernan et al. *Experimental Gerontology* (2011). PMID: 20883771

26 Ye et al. *Aging* (2010). PMID: 20606248

27 Giordani et al. *Diabetes and Metabolism* (2014). PMID: 24439268

28 Dansinger et al. *JAMA* (2005). PMID: 15632335

29 Chao et al. *The Journal of Clinical Investigation* (2021). PMID: 33393504

30 Churuangsuk et al. *Obesity Reviews* (2018). PMID: 30194696

31 Gardner et al. *JAMA* (2018). PMID: 29466592

32 Foster et al. *The New England Journal of Medicine* (2003). PMID: 12761365

33 Wang et al. *JAMA* (2021). PMID: 34374722

34 Schnabel et al. *JAMA Internal Medicine* (2019). PMID: 30742202

35 Askari et al. *International Journal of Obesity* (2020). PMID: 32796919

36 Hull et al. *European Journal of Nutrition* (2015). PMID: 25182142

37 Mohammadi-Sartang et al. *Obesity Reviews* (2017). PMID: 28635182
38 Kondo et al. *Bioscience, Biotechnology and Biochemistry* (2009). PMID: 19661687
39 Chao et al. *The Journal of Clinical Investigation* (2021). PMID: 33393504
40 Mancini et al. *The American Journal of Medicine* (2016). PMID: 26721635
41 Smethers et al. *The Medical Clinics of North America* (2018). PMID: 29156179
42 Darmadi-Blackberry et al. *Asia Pacific Journal of Clinical Nutrition* (2004). PMID: 15228991
43 Bao et al. *The New England Journal of Medicine* (2013). PMID: 24256379
44 Tremblay et al. *The International Journal of Behavioral Nutrition and Physical Activity* (2017). PMID: 28599680
45 Biswas et al. *Annals of Internal Medicine* (2015). PMID: 25599350
46 Ekelund et al. *Lancet* (2016). PMID: 27475271
47 Chang et al. *Journal of the American Heart Association* (2020). PMID: 32063113
48 Chang et al. *Canadian Journal of Diabetes* (2020). PMID: 33279098
49 Washburn et al. *PLoS One* (2014). PMID: 25333384
50 Ruegsegger et al. *Cold Spring Harbor Perspectives in Medicine* (2018). PMID: 28507196
51 Jakicic et al. *International Journal of Obesity and Related Metabolic Disorders* (1995). PMID: 7550521
52 Ahmadi et al. *European Heart Journal* (2022). PMID: 36302460
53 Swift et al. *Progress in Cardiovascular Diseases* (2018). PMID: 30003901
54 Wing et al. *The American Journal of Clinical Nutrition* (2005). PMID: 16002825
55 Swift et al. *Progress in Cardiovascular Diseases* (2018). PMID: 30003901
56 Su et al. *PLoS One* (2019). PMID: 30689632
57 Donnelly et al. *Obesity* (2013). PMID: 23592678
58 Swift et al. *Progress in Cardiovascular Diseases* (2018). PMID: 30003901
59 Willis et al. *Journal of Applied Physiology* (2012). PMID: 23019316
60 Church et al. *JAMA* (2010). PMID: 21098771
61 Momma et al. *British Journal of Sports Medicine* (2022). PMID: 35228201
62 Willis et al. *Journal of Applied Physiology* (2012). PMID: 23019316
63 D'Aurea et al. *Brazilian Journal of Psychiatry* (2019). PMID: 30328967
64 Kovacevic et al. *Sleep Medicine Reviews* (2018). PMID: 28919335

65 Gordan et al. *JAMA Psychiatry* (2018). PMID: 29800984
66 Gordan et al. *Sports Medicine* (2017). PMID: 28819746
67 Hashida et al. *Journal of Hepatology* (2017). PMID: 27639843
68 Shiroma et al. *Medicine and Science in Sports and Exercise* (2017). PMID: 27580152
69 Nery et al. *Brazilian Journal of Physical Therapy* (2017). PMID: 28728958
70 Naci et al. *British Journal of Sports Medicine* (2019). PMID: 30563873
71 Hollings et al. *European Journal of Preventive Cardiology* (2017). PMID: 28578612
72 Kodama et al. *JAMA* (2009). PMID: 19454641
73 Westcott. *Current Sports Medicine Reports* (2012). PMID: 19454641
74 Taheri et al. *PLoS Medicine* (2004). PMID: 15602591
75 Lv et al. *Appetite* (2018). PMID: 29447996
76 Heath et al. *Accident: Analysis and Prevention* (2012). PMID: 22239934
77 Hogenkamp et al. *Psychoneuroendocrinology* (2013). PMID: 23428257
78 Capers et al. *Obesity Reviews* (2015). PMID: 26098388
79 Chaput et al. *International Journal of Obesity* (2012). PMID: 21654631
80 Nedeltcheva et al. *Annals of Internal Medicine* (2010). PMID: 20921542
81 Taheri et al. *PLoS Medicine* (2004). PMID: 15602591
82 Shi et al. *Sleep Medicine Reviews* (2018). PMID: 28890168
83 Ma et al. *JAMA Newtork Open* (2020). PMID: 32955572
84 Wang et al. *BMC Psychiatry* (2019). PMID: 31623600
85 Woznica et al. *Sleep Medicine Reviews* (2015). PMID: 25454672
86 Roberts et al. *Sleep* (2014). PMID: 24497652
87 Pires et al. *Sleep Medicine* (2016). PMID: 27810176
88 Tochikubo et al. *Hypertension* (1996). PMID: 8641742
89 King et al. *JAMA* (2008). PMID: 19109114
90 Fernandez-Mendoza et al. *Journal of the American Heart Association* (2019). PMID: 31575322
91 Koren et al. *Metabolism* (2018). PMID: 29630921
92 Wittert. *Current Opinion in Endocrinology, Diabetes and Obesity* (2014). PMID: 24739309
93 Chen et al. *Environment International* (2020). PMID: 31830732
94 Lim et al. *PLoS One* (2016). PMID: 27870902
95 Queiroz et al. *Sleep Health* (2020). PMID: 32448713
96 Holding et al. *Journal of Sleep Research* (2019). PMID: 31006920
97 Tomiyama et al. *Annual Review of Psychology* (2019). PMID: 29927688

98   Chao et al. *Obesity* (2017). PMID: 28349668
99   Spencer et al. *Stress* (2011). PMID: 21294656
100 Scott et al. *Current Obesity Reports* (2012). PMID: 22943039
101 Leger et al. *Stress Health* (2020). PMID: 32472738
102 Black et al. *JAMA Internal Medicine* (2015). PMID: 25686304
103 Zeiden et al. *Consciousness and Cognition* (2010). PMID: 20363650
104 Rogers et al. *Obesity Reviews* (2017). PMID: 27862826
105 Goyal et al. *JAMA Internal Medicine* (2014). PMID: 24395196
106 Katterman et al. *Eating Behaviors* (2014). PMID: 24854804
107 Lyubomirsky et al. *Psychological Bulletin* (2005). PMID: 16351326
108 Diener et al. *Perspectives on Psychological Science* (2018). PMID: 29592642
109 Emmons et al. *Journal of Personality and Social Psychology* (2003). PMID: 12585811
110 Whillans et al. *Health Psychology* (2016). PMID: 26867038
111 Saxon et al. *Obesity* (2019). PMID: 31603630
112 Haddock et al. *International Journal of Obesity and Related Metabolic Disorders* (2002). PMID: 11850760
113 Monro et al. *BMJ* (1968). PMID: 15508204
114 Khera et al. *JAMA* (2016). PMID: 27299618
115 Khera et al. *JAMA* (2016). PMID: 27299618
116 Apovian et al. *Obesity* (2013). PMID: 23408728
117 Khera et al. *JAMA* (2016). PMID: 27299618
118 Pi-Sunyer et al. *The New England Journal of Medicine* (2015). PMID: 26132939
119 Wilding et al. *The New England Journal of Medicine* (2021). PMID: 33567185
120 Brownley et al. *Annals of Internal Medicine* (2016). PMID: 27367316
121 Yerevanian et al. *Current Obesity Reports* (2019). PMID: 30874963
122 Holman et al. *The New England Journal of Medicine* (2008). PMID: 18784090
123 DeFronzo et al. *The New England Journal of Medicine* (1995). PMID: 7623902
124 de Silva et al. *BMC Psychiatry* (2016). PMID: 27716110
125 Ribola et al. *European Review for Medical and Pharmacological Sciences* (2017). PMID: 28121337
126 Min et al. *Diabetes Therapy* (2021). PMID: 33325008
127 Frias et al. *The New England Journal of Medicine* (2021). PMID: 34170647
128 Hollander et al. *Diabetes Care* (2017). PMID: 28289041
129 Lau et al. *Lancet* (2021). PMID: 34798060
130 Enebo et al. *Lancet* (2021). PMID: 33894838
131 Srivastava et al. *Nature Reviews: Endocrinology* (2018). PMID: 29027993

132 Elkins et al. *Obesity Surgery* (2005). PMID: 15946436
133 Arterburn et al. *JAMA* (2020). PMID: 32870301
134 Sjostrom et al. *The New England Journal of Medicine* (2007). PMID: 17715408
135 Adams et al. *The New England Journal of Medicine* (2007). PMID: 17715409
136 Arterburn et al. *JAMA* (2020). PMID: 32870301
137 Lee et al. *Annals of Surgery* (2021). PMID: 31693504
138 Gu et al. *BMC Surgery* (2020). PMID: 32050953
139 Climent et al. *Journal of Hypertension* (2020). PMID: 31633582
140 Wiggins et al. *Obesity Surgery* (2019). PMID: 30591985
141 Arterburn et al. *JAMA* (2020). PMID: 32870301
142 Arterburn et al. *JAMA* (2018). PMID: 29340659

Chapter 5

How can we be successful

It would be nice if we were able to help our patients by simply telling them what to do and giving them a medication. 'Mr. Jones please eat less, move more, sleep well, reduce your stress, and take this medication and you should be all set.' Unfortunately, it does not work that way. Step 1 is to see if weight is of any concern to them. If not on their radar at the moment, move on to the next subject. In future visits, try to relate current medical conditions or lab results to their weight, in hopes of opening their mind to the possibility of weight loss. Telling someone to lose weight never works; they must want to lose weight themselves. If they are worried about their weight, then the next step is to determine if they are ready to make changes now. Ask them on a scale of 1–10 how important it is to lose weight. If the answer is 8 or above, then we can start talking about a weight loss plan. You have learned what can help with weight loss in the previous chapter. But knowing is only half the battle. The cornerstone of weight loss management is behavioral therapy. Give your patients skillpower, and do not let them rely on willpower. This may seem daunting to you as that has never been a part of your provider training. But as you will soon find out, these skills include a lot of common sense and can be done in an efficient manner at every medical office visit; with practice, you can be a master of behavioral therapy.

COGNITIVE BEHAVIORAL THERAPY

The following are cognitive behavioral strategies that can be applied to your patients. The therapeutic relationship and agenda setting involve tasks that you, the healthcare provider, can work

DOI: 10.1201/9781003371595-5

on to help the patient at each visit. The rest are specific skills that can be discussed with a patient and then used to create action plans (formerly known as 'homework'). For example, let's say you are doing a follow-up on a chronic medical condition such as dyslipidemia. You ask about compliance with the statin, order labs, calculate the ASCVD risk score, determine if a Coronary Artery Calcium (CAC) score is needed, and then mention how consistent healthy lifestyle habits (specifically, more foods from the Portfolio diet such as beans, lentils, flaxseed, nuts, eggplant, okra, and oatmeal) will go a long way to helping improve the cholesterol levels. In the last 2 minutes of the visit, you can discuss one of the below cognitive behavioral strategies and ask the patient to apply it for the next 4 weeks or until the next office visit. You encourage the patient to complete this task by saying 'knowing what to do to improve your health is not enough unfortunately. It is the consistency of the habit that matters. To make healthy habits more consistent and a natural part of your daily routine, there are specific strategies that can help, and this is one of them.'

Therapeutic relationship

The therapeutic relationship is the concept that the provider–patient interaction on its own can influence positive health outcomes. Not all interactions will be positive. But if there is respect and trust in the relationship, there is a good chance every encounter can be productive. An example of a way to build this relationship is to remember to write down in the chart if something significant happened to your patient in his or her personal life such as the loss of a pet or a promotion at work. At future visits, when you randomly bring these topics up, it will trigger an emotion in your patient that will pay dividends down the road, such as compliance with a medication you recommend. Other ways to enhance the therapeutic relationship include having a comfortable waiting room, offering patients water, eye contact (not staring at your laptop), and smiling. A unique way to connect to your patients that also breaks the negative thoughts the brain is wired to focus on is to ask them this specific question during the office visit, 'Tell me something good that happened to you last week?'. You can also share something good that happened to you to get the ball rolling. This one simple act can change the entire relationship you have with your patient.

Agenda setting

We healthcare providers have no time to waste. We dread the infamous patient who is about to leave and then casually says, 'Can you refill my asthma inhaler, the red one, and then look at the mole on my back?'. Set an agenda right from the start and never be surprised again. It is a remarkable time-saving strategy. For example, you can say, 'Today we will be discussing your new medication and following up on your eating habits. In the brief time we have today is there something else you would like to talk about?'. You may be afraid to do this in fear of opening up Pandora's box. That is understandable. But it makes the patient feel heard and makes the visit go by smoothly and efficiently. This strategy is used by cognitive behavioral therapists at all their sessions. Make it a part of your office visit strategy.

Self-monitoring

This is the most reliable technique to help with weight loss. In a systematic review by Ramage et al. in 2014, 92% of successful weight loss interventions included self-monitoring.[1] Self-monitoring is simply creating awareness of all things that can affect weight loss. The obvious things to monitor are food intake and physical activity. Other less obvious items to monitor include sleep quantity and quality, emotions during the day (and specifically before food intake), and stress level. A good way to be aware of these things is by journaling. This may seem like a cumbersome task, but time and time again leads to results.[2] National programs like Weight Watchers, Noom, and Jenny Craig use self-monitoring. Take advantage of modern technology with apps and wearables that take the effort out of self-monitoring. Ask your patient to get a new notebook and at least monitor all the above for 4 days every month. This can be done once a week or 4 days in a row, whatever the patient prefers. This will help the patient get back on track every month before habits turn for the worse.

Goal setting

Your patients Hgb A1c comes back at 7.2, and they are already on metformin. You may quickly mention that they need to cut down on sugary snacks, eat more vegetables, and exercise more. The patient agrees with you and on to the next patient you go. Three to

6 months later, the patient comes back with a similar Hgb A1c and you start thinking of additional medications to control the blood sugar. To help your patient fix the root problems, the SMART technique may be useful. It takes a lot less time than you would think. SMART was created by George Duran, Arthur Miller, and James Cunningham in 1981. Going back to that first office visit, suppose you said 'I believe you can reach a Hgb A1c of below 7 as this will lower your chances of diabetic complications in the future.' We know processed foods such as desserts, sugar-sweetened beverages, and packaged snacks can worsen diabetes, while increasing fiber can improve your blood sugar control. Let's focus on making one or two specific changes in your eating habits. Of all the snacks/desserts you have, is there one you would like to reduce? Also, let's pick a specific fiber-rich vegetable, say pinto beans or kale or eggplant and see if we can incorporate that into the diet more often. After a quick discussion with the patient, you can summarize the visit by saying 'over the next 4 weeks you will have only two cans of soda versus the current six cans a week as goal number one, and you will have pinto beans 4 days a week versus occasionally as the second goal.' This simple act of giving a specific goal to the patient can jumpstart a healthy lifestyle revolution for the patient.

Let's go through another example. You want to help your patient have less alcohol.

Specific – Just saying you want them to have less alcohol really won't help them be successful. Instead, negotiate with your patient and come up with specific goals. For example, having alcohol twice a week (versus everyday), maximum of two drinks on the day you decide to drink (versus four or more), wine only (versus wine or beer or liquor), 6 ounces (versus a 'tall' glass), only with dinner (versus anytime), and on Friday and Saturday nights (versus any random night).

Measurable – You decided two 6-ounce glasses of wine on Friday/Saturday nights with dinner. All of that can be measured. If you had just decided 'less' wine, it really would not be measurable.

Achievable – Your patient can drink less alcohol. A goal of swimming the Indian Ocean on the other hand may not be achievable.

Relevant and Realistic – Always stop and think to make sure the behavior you are trying to change is relevant to your patient's goal. Secondly, make sure the goal is realistic. This is where understanding where your patient is on the transtheoretical model of change is important. Knowing the different stages is not as important as knowing how to apply that information. In that regard, you can ask one simple question. On a scale of 1–10, how confident are you in the goal we made today? If the answer is below 8, they are less likely to succeed. In that case, ask them what stopped them from saying 8 or 9; what barriers do they perceive? This will be paramount information for your patient's success.

Timed – This is something people always forget. Always put a time frame to the goal you are setting; otherwise, it may seem a bit daunting to the patient to make a change that is forever. For the specific goal you made above, you decide your patient will stick to it for 4 weeks only. After 4 weeks, tell the patient to reassess. If the patient was successful, tell them to pat themselves on the back and keep going. If they were not successful, tell them that is the perfect time to use their problem-solving skills. For example, if they did not stick to two nights a week of drinking and instead drank four times a week, tell the patient, first, they improved from before so that is excellent. Secondly, after problem solving, they may have figured out that it was difficult to drink only on the weekend because of after-work social gatherings every Tuesday and Thursday. This is good news. Because of this goal-setting behavior, we now have a specific target of helping the patient with drinking during social gatherings. Helping the patient through this task may unlock the secret to their success. Good luck!

Motivation

Motivation is the single most important factor when it comes to trying to change any behavior. Some behavioral experts may argue that statement. Motivation is something that may take several visits to figure out in your patient, but be persistent, and when you find what makes your patient tick, find ways to bring it up in conversations at almost every visit. Motivation can be broken down into three levels as follows:

Long-term motivation – These are the deep-rooted reasons why everyone tries to aspire to be as healthy as possible. Examples include 'I want to live a long life so that I can spend time with my grandchildren,' 'I want to avoid diabetes,' and 'I want to look my best for my partner.' The problem with this type of motivation is that you don't think of these reasons in the moment you are about to do an unhelpful behavior such as eating a bag of chips or working long hours at work or going to bed late at night. Patients will succeed in their behavior change if you remind them of their long-term motivations. You can say, 'I recommend writing down on a small piece of paper, your top ten reasons for wanting to be healthy and keeping it somewhere you can see daily like the fridge or your nightstand. Initially, it should be read every day.'

Short-term motivation – These are rewards or reinforcements that are 2–4 weeks away. You can use almost anything as a motivational tool. Examples include 'if I reduce my meat intake for the next 2 weeks, I will buy that shirt I've wanted for a while' or 'if I walk every day for 20 minutes for the next 2 weeks, I will watch that movie I've been dying to see.' These short-term motivations work like a charm, but the key is to constantly find innovative ways to reward yourself.

Immediate motivation – These are positive affirmations that your patient can say to themselves right after they complete a healthy habit. Examples include 'I went to the gym just now, I am awesome' or 'I avoided the cookies in the lunchroom today, I am awesome.' Tell your patients that this skill may feel awkward at first but over time becomes a habit. Your patient already talks to themselves all the time. It just happens to be negative comments. Such as 'I shouldn't have had that extra slice of pizza, I have no willpower' or, 'I got stressed at work and ate a box of cookies. I'm so stupid'. Reverse this trend, and teach your patients to be positive to themselves.

Accountability

Studies like the Look AHEAD trial confirm that those subjects that attended their group or one-on-one sessions more regularly did better than those that did not when it comes to weight loss.[3] Those sessions kept the patients accountable. When a patient knows there is an appointment with a health provider coming up, they get a bit more motivated or focused on their healthy habits closer to the appointment. If you have the luxury of seeing patients weekly, then that on its own will lead to success for your patients. Unfortunately, that is not realistic for most providers. As a result, the key point here is to let your patients know they can use any health or wellness provider as an accountability measure and even their family and friends. This is a major ingredient to success. For example, over the span of a few months, if a patient has appointments with their primary care provider, obesity medicine specialist, chiropractor, massage therapist, and say a yoga instructor, then each of those visits can be used as an accountability tool to help keep the patient focused. All you must do is tell the patient to think of those appointments in that manner.

Problem solving

Your patient is already a great problem solver. They have been problem solving their entire lives. Every time they have faced an obstacle professionally or socially, they have figured out a way forward. That has brought them to this point. You are now asking them to apply their problem-solving experience to their own healthy lifestyle habit goals. They need to sit down and schedule out time in their day to figure out how they can incorporate more healthy habits into their daily routine. But you have to tell them to do that; otherwise, no one really carves out time for themselves to figure things out. If they are struggling (which is almost 100% of humankind), then they have the luxury of having you on their side. You can problem solve together. A useful technique for problem solving that is evidence based and created by Gabrielle Oettingen is called WOOP (Wish, Outcome, Obstacle, Plan).[4] Let's use this in an example.

You have been trying to get your patient to walk more as part of their weight loss or healthy living plan. You used the SMART strategy to create a very specific goal of walking outside for 15 minutes, 6 days a week every morning. Over the past month, your patient has not reached their goal. You decide today to figure this out, and you use the WOOP technique (I use it slightly differently from the original form).

<u>W</u>ish – This is the larger goal your patient has. For example, 'I want to lose 20 lbs' or 'I want to live a long healthy life.'

<u>O</u>utcome – This is the specific task of concern that is trying to be completed in order to inch toward that larger goal or 'wish.' In this case, I want to walk a minimum of 15 minutes 6 days a week.

<u>O</u>bstacle – This can be an external or internal obstacle. External is 'rain or cold weather prevents me from walking.' Internal obstacle is a negative-thought process that gets in the way of achieving the goal. For example, 'I feel lazy in the morning' or '15 minutes is too little, and if I can't walk 60 minutes, there is no point in walking at all.'

<u>P</u>lan – This is the fun part. This is where you brainstorm. First thought that may enter your mind is how am I letting the weather control my fate. I am just making excuses here. If I just change my mindset (this is called cognitive restructuring), I will find a way

to walk every day. Then you plan for those obstacles by saying to yourself, IF it rains, THEN I will ___ (blank space). Fill in that blank space with whatever works for you. Examples include I will drive to the mall and walk there, I will use the treadmill in the gym in the building, I will walk later in the day when it is not raining, or I will simply enjoy the rain and get a raincoat or umbrella. A point to keep in mind here is that the patient is the expert of themselves and not you. So rely on the patient for the actual solutions. That makes this process feel less burdensome from the provider perspective.

As you get more comfortable with WOOP, it can be used at any office visit and take up a few minutes of your time.

Stimulus control

What makes obesity management difficult is the unique life your patient lives and has lived. Which specific triggers lead to unhelpful habits needs to be explored by you and the patient; otherwise, the best weight loss plan in the world can be sabotaged right from the start. Triggers can be broken down into four major categories:

1. Social Triggers – A birthday party. Thanksgiving holiday. Meeting up with a friend for dinner. Anniversary. Major sporting event. Social gatherings and the expectation to enjoy oneself with food and alcohol will never stop.
2. Environmental Triggers – The smell from the local Krispy Kreme. The cookies in the kitchen that are left on the counter. The bar that you always drive by on the way back from work. The commercial on TV about a snickers bar.
3. Mental Triggers – Thinking of food. Reading about food. Listening to a friend talk about food.
4. Emotional Triggers – A hard day at work leading to wanting a glass of wine. Feeling bored so reaching for the bag of chips. Feeling lonely, isolated, or depressed and thus making it easier to enjoy dessert.

Teach your patient these triggers. Just awareness of them can help fix some of them. Others will need more work, and applying the WOOP technique to problem solve is a good start. A good strategy to help in these 'trigger' moments (for example, a patient is sad and is about to open the fridge door) is the ABCD technique. 'A' stands for Awareness. The patient being more mindful of these moments will go a long way toward success. 'B' stands for Breathing.

Take one full minute to take slow deep breaths. 'C' stands for cold water. Slowly drink half a glass of cold water. Finally, 'D' stands for Distractions. Ask the patient to write down ten ways they can distract themselves in these moments. Examples include going for a walk, texting a friend, reading a book, starting a TV show, etc.

Social support

Extrinsic motivation from family and friends is a successful strategy. The problem is family and friends can also sabotage a great game plan. Whether it's a husband opening a bag of chips while watching TV or a friend encouraging one more drink at a party, these can be difficult situations. Therefore, finding friends and family that are supportive is paramount. At the office visit, ask your patient to identify specific friends or family members that will support her healthy lifestyle journey. Once these people are identified, ask the patient to write down ways they can support her. Examples include workout partners, healthy eating coworkers to have lunch with, or weekly phone calls with a friend for accountability and cheering on the patient (Figure 5.1).

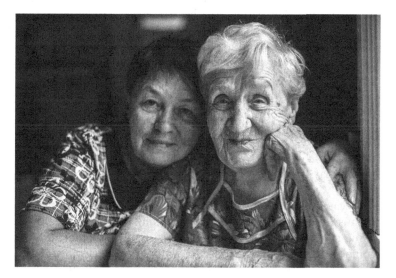

Figure 5.1   Do not underestimate the power of social connections in your patient's weight loss efforts. Ask your patient about who they spend time with the most and have them use them for accountability. Plus, you never know if spending more time with friends or family will allow for stress to go down and weight to melt right off.

Cognitive restructuring

People have certain ingrained thought patterns that work against them and the goals they have. If these cognitive distortions can be changed, it may get easier to stick to goals. This is the basic idea behind cognitive restructuring. Of course, this is easier said than done, as these thought processes are connected to core beliefs which have been a part of the patient since childhood probably. As a physician, you may not have the time to work through the cognitive distortions as thoroughly as a CBT therapist, but you can at least be aware of the common cognitive distortions. You can then make the patient aware of these 'unhelpful thoughts' so that the patient can attempt to problem solve around them or seek the help of a therapist.

The biggest cognitive error to keep in mind is 'All or None' thinking. It is very common among patients seeking help for weight loss. A patient has a slice of cake at a birthday party and because it is not part of the plan, they feel guilt, and this leads to having two glasses of regular coke, two slices of pizza, and a bag of chips. Now patient comes home, and they overgeneralize and judge themselves to be weak based on one single isolated event. This now leads to days to weeks of unhealthy eating, and because they feel like they are off the plan, the exercise has ceased as well. This cycle of events you will see, and when you do, please stop and discuss it. Over time, a patient can learn to have a piece of cake and immediately afterward go back to healthy eating without even thinking about it.

Fortune telling is another cognitive distortion. This is when a patient already predicts the outcome of a certain strategy or plan you are trying to make with them and usually the outcome they are thinking is negative. This prediction is not based on any specific facts or likelihood. If you can point that out in a kind and subtle way, it may convince your patient to give the plan an honest effort.

Finally, the 'health halo' cognitive distortion is a personal favorite because majority of us fall for this. We walk into Subway, and because we already feel like we are doing something healthy by going to Subway versus say another fast-food restaurant, we overcompensate by getting a soda and chips. The biggest health halo effect comes after exercise, specifically walking. You go to the mall and walk more than usual or walk all day while on vacation in a foreign city. In both situations, people are inclined to eat bigger portions and more processed carbohydrate-heavy foods because they feel like they burned a lot of calories with their activity. Unfortunately, it never equates. You can give your patients the example that if they jogged for 45 minutes and at the end of the jog had a black coffee with a muffin, it would leave them at net-zero calories burned basically.

Education

Knowledge is what will get your patient to go above and beyond for themselves. An assumption we all make as physicians is thinking that certain lifestyle habits are just not possible for the patient. That they would never stop drinking alcohol or start running every day for 30 minutes. This is a costly error in judgment. An older lady who has never exercised in her life, loves to cook for her family, and has English as a second language may seem like an impossible candidate for making lifestyle changes. But you will be pleasantly surprised at what they can do after gaining some knowledge. There is only so much you can impart during an office visit, so you must rely on outside sources. Create a patient handout that lists credible sources of health information that you endorse and update it yearly. Examples may include other health professionals in the community. Ask your patient to create a circle of trusted experts such as chiropractor, physical therapists, nutritionist, massage therapist, and yoga instructor. Remind the patient to take advantage of these experts by constantly asking questions at every visit. Recommend podcasts such as Obesity: A disease from the Obesity Medicine Association and Nutrition Facts with Dr. Gregor. Introduce them to websites from prominent organizations like the Obesity Action Coalition, American Heart Association, etc. Bibliotherapy is improving one's health through reading of books like *The Obesity Code*, *The Circadian Code*, *The Longevity Diet*, etc. Follow experts on social media like Dr. Mark Hyman from the Cleveland Clinic.

Assertiveness training

Learning to say NO. There will always be situations where the patient encounters unwanted calories from unexpected (and expected) sources. The patient is not obliged to have a piece of cake when it's the boss's birthday at work. You can show them how to say no. Ask the patient to spend 1 month making note of all instances where someone else offered a drink or food with calories. It can be an entertaining and fun task for the patient. It forces the patient to be more aware of these situations. This awareness on its own will lead to the patient understanding the significant influence of the people around them, and they will naturally have less calories this way. But there is one other task that will further help the patient. Ask the patient for a week or two to say NO to all these instances of being offered a food or drink with calories. Not an easy task for patients. In many cultures, it can be a big sign of disrespect when saying no to food or snacks being offered in their homes. These are the difficult situations you must ask your patient to think about for success to occur.

Relapse prevention strategies

A lapse is a temporary setback in the new lifestyle habit changes a patient is making, while a relapse is a more permanent setback. It takes 4 weeks to begin a new habit, 2 months to make it more automatic, and 1–2 years to make it permanent. During this time, lapses are a normal part of the change process. This information will help prevent your patient from feeling guilty and hopeless when they fall into a bad habit for one moment or 1 day. This is important because what usually occurs after a single lapse is the feeling of 'oh well' and then comes overindulgence for the rest of the day or week or month. Relapse prevention strategies are basically problem-solving sessions where you anticipate situations where lapses may occur and figure out creative solutions.

MOTIVATIONAL INTERVIEWING

Motivational interviewing is a style of conversation with your patient that leads to helpful changes in behavior that lead to positive health outcomes. A meta-analysis in 2011 included 12 RCTs and examined the effect of motivational interviewing on weight loss. It showed a significant weight loss effect of about 3 lbs.[5] In a 2021 systematic review and meta-analysis by Makin et al., no effect on weight was found. But there are many limitations to studying the specific effects of motivational interviewing on weight loss as you can imagine.[6] This style is one of collaborating with the patient and giving them autonomy over the decisions that affect their health. This contrasts with simply telling the patient what to do, which seems like an archaic way of practicing medicine. You are the expert in medicine, but the patient is the expert in themselves. Together health decisions can be made that the patient will be compliant with, mostly because they decided and not you, the provider. This way of speaking to the patient will bear fruit in many aspects of medicine, but a clear example is in adherence to medications. It is mind boggling how often patients do not take their medications. We physicians are just as horrible in following up with our patients to ensure compliance. This is highlighted in patients with recent acute coronary syndromes. You would think 100% of patients would be on statins afterward. Yet real-world data from cardiology clinics tell us that only 50% of patients remain on statins 6–12 months later and even less on the recommended high-intensity statins. This example is from cardiology clinics and after a heart attack! There are probably a myriad of reasons why statin use is not 100% here including statin-associated side effects. But if the patients were told in the hospital and at follow-up visits, of the data showing the incidence of recurrent major adverse cardiac events in patient on statins versus off statins, it would signify to the patient the importance of sticking to their medication regimen. To further help in this regard, if we used motivational interviewing, we would understand the barriers the patient has in their minds to this new medication they are being asked to take after a heart attack. We can then help the patient with any uncertainties right away, and this would solidify our confidence that the patient truly understands the grave importance of taking a statin (or PCSK9i for that matter) after a myocardial infarction and will be compliant moving forward (Figure 5.2).

The basic tenets of motivational interviewing include giving the patient *autonomy* to make their own decisions after collaborating with them on discussing the risks and benefits of the situation, showing *empathy*, developing *discrepancy*, supporting *self-efficacy*, and *rolling with resistance.*

It all starts with rolling with resistance. Your patient will resist most of the amazing evidence you know can help them. This can be very frustrating. It would be very easy to show that frustration by judging the patient as a failure and noncompliant. But where does that get you and more importantly, where does that get your patient. When presented with resistance from the patient, the first thing to do is simply listen to them. Showing the patient that you

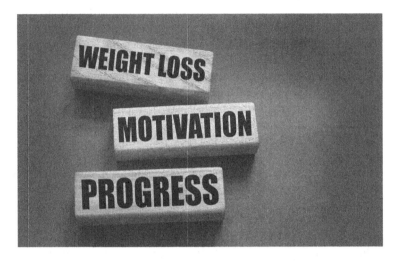

Figure 5.2   Motivation is something you will hear a lot when it comes to behavior change and weight loss. In the office, if you are genuinely kind to your patient and tell them you care about them, you will be surprised how powerful a motivation can be for your patient. Try it today.

hear their concerns goes a long way with them (empathy). This act of listening on its own may make the patient less resistant. But to really get your patient to see the other side, reinforce the risk/benefit ratio and highlight the patient's current actions and how it differs from their own desired goals (developing discrepancy). Once they see this and soften their stance on changing, pounce on this 'change talk' by boosting their confidence in their ability to succeed in this behavior change (self-efficacy). A great way to enhance confidence is to take examples from the patient's own past where they overcame a challenge. If they can become a CEO or a lawyer, they can be successful in a single task like eating within a certain window of time. After boosting their confidence, it's a good idea to summarize the goals you and the patient have decided together.

POSITIVE PSYCHOLOGY

Positive psychology is the study of the strengths and virtues that allow individuals to thrive. Dr. Martin Seligman is a leading voice in the field of positive psychology and created the five pillars (acronym PERMA): Positive emotion (the ability to be optimistic and the ability to view the past, present, and future in a positive fashion), Engagement (being fully absorbed into the present moment with a 'blissful immersion' that stretches intelligence, skill, and emotional capacity), Relationships (one of the most important aspects of life are positive social connections with other humans emotionally and physically), Meaning (having a purpose for why one is on earth is important to living a life of fulfillment and happiness), and Accomplishments (having ambition and accomplishing realistic goals produces a sense of satisfaction, pride, and fulfillment).[7] Using the pillars and the principles of positive psychology, you can create tasks that enhance each area. Examples can include asking patients to do a gratitude journal, volunteer for something they are passionate about, and spending more time in nature (Figure 5.3).

What is the connection of positive psychology to weight loss? These tasks enhance emotional well-being. This directly

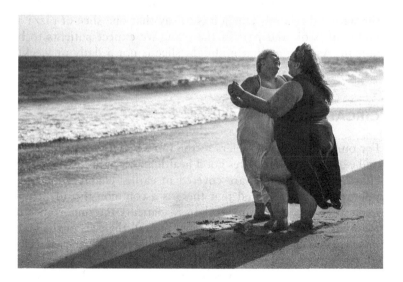

Figure 5.3   In the end, the number on the scale truly does not matter. What matters is striving for good health so that you can enjoy life and your purpose for as long as possible. That extension of quality of life is what we are striving to achieve. Tell your patients that. Otherwise, they get bogged down by that number on the scale, and it can hinder their weight loss efforts.

improves health by changing the physiology in the body such as change in cortisol levels and normalizing dopamine responses in the brain. But the biggest impact is that as patients start to feel better about themselves, they are more likely to follow your recommendations such as eating one more serving of fruit a day or spending 20 more minutes on a treadmill. In a study, negative emotions mainly predicted the intake of unhealthy food, whereas positive emotions predicted physical activity (intention and behavior).[8]

A key skill to remember here is to always ask the patient to focus on what they did well since their last visit and to continuously point to all the good habits they are currently doing. This is because the human mind is wired to focus on the negative. Kind of like an ancestral mechanism that protects us from anything bad happening to us. A patient can be doing many things well during a certain week, but the one misstep they made, such as going to bed late one night and having a midnight pizza slice, is what they focus on. If that becomes the focus, it can lead to negative feelings of guilt which can easily turn the patient down the wrong direction. Our job is to say that one slice of pizza at midnight is ok and part of the plan. We expect patients to be human. As long as that midnight slice is not a daily or weekly event!

CIRCADIAN RHYTHM

For our purposes, this refers to the timing of food intake, sleep, and exercise that promotes good health and weight loss. The specific recommendations are covered in earlier chapters, but it is important to understand that there is a common thread. It will make it easier for you to explain to patients the importance of these lifestyle habit changes. Simply put, all the cells of the body have their own internal clock. This includes heart muscle cells, liver cells, and pancreatic cells. If you take an individual cell from any organ in the body and observe it in a lab, it will go about its cellular processes in a rhythmic manner. Now, there is also a master clock in the body in the suprachiasmatic nucleus located in the hypothalamus. Both the master clock and the individual clocks in every cell have a 24 rhythmic cycle that mimics the day–night cycle. This means hormones and other chemical messengers are released in a rhythmic pattern throughout the day. If you know when these hormones are higher and when they are lower, then you can appreciate the physiology and take advantage of it. This is what we are trying to do. When you tell a patient to have their carbohydrates earlier in the day, you are basically telling them that their body will be more efficient in processing those calories during the day because the hormones are optimal for doing that. When the patient has an evening snack after dinner, or a midnight craving satisfied with a bowl of cereal, they are going against their circadian rhythm. The food timing on its own, regardless of the calories, will lead to poor health outcomes if repeated consistently and prevent their goal of weight loss. Once again, all calories are not made equal.

This is a burgeoning field of science, and we are just beginning to understand the complexity. For example, studies done in rodents show if two groups of rats are given the same number of calories, but one group has those calories when they are supposed to sleep, they gain a significant amount of weight.[9] This has translated into human studies on time-restricted feeding as discussed in previous chapters. We can also see the ill effects of going against our own circadian rhythm when we study night-shift workers—a 57% increase in risk of metabolic syndrome,[10] an 18% increased risk of atrial fibrillation, and a 22% increased risk of coronary heart disease.[11] In a 2020 cross-sectional study by Brum et al., night-shift workers had a three times higher risk of abdominal obesity than day-shift workers.[12] This is unfortunate since 18% of the US work force do not work a regular day shift.[13] This percentage is similar in other countries as well. What can you do to help your night-shift-working patients? First is educating them on the dangers to their health. Then I would have an honest conversation with the patient and suggest that if it at all was under their control to change to day shift, that you would recommend that not only for their weight loss goals but overall health and longevity. As this may not be an option, there are some changes your patient can make to help such as having their dinner before their shift and no calories during their shift, plus optimizing all the other aspects of care discussed in the book earlier. Night-shift workers are fighting an uphill battle, but at least, they have you helping them in every way you can.

CASE STUDY CONTINUED

Martha got her Semaglutide (Wegovy) approved and has been on it for 3 weeks. She returns today to discuss.

Dr. C: Good afternoon, Martha. How are you doing?

M: I'm great. Thank you for asking.

Dr. C: Looks like you have been on the Wegovy for 3 weeks now, any side effects of nausea or constipation?

M: I do feel a bit nauseated the first couple of days after I take the injection, but it is nothing severe. I am still able to go about my day.

Dr. C: Well, I am glad the side effects are minimal. You mentioned the nausea within the first few days. A positive way to look at this is that the nausea indicates that the medication is working. Of course, I do not want you to be nauseated all the time. Things that can help reduce nausea are smaller portions, eating slowly and not lying down after meals/snacks. I also usually tell patients to take the medication on a Thursday so that maximum impact of the medication can be used to help curb appetite on weekends. A time when patients struggle a bit more. You can think about using it in that way as well.

M: I think I might do that. That is good to know.

Dr. C: You are currently on the 0.25 mg dose still so I would not expect significant weight loss yet, but I have had patients lose weight during the initial month. You seem to be in that category as well. As you have lost 5 lbs already. Congratulations.

M: Thanks Dr. C, but I did nothing. It's just the medication.

Dr. C: I would beg to differ. Honestly, this is an important point to make here. I need you to give yourself the credit. You did this. This is not easy, and the medication helps for sure. But in the end, it is you making the daily changes and sticking to it as best as you can. That hard work should not go unnoticed.

M: Thank you.

Dr. C: I will go ahead and refill the Wegovy at the next highest dose of 0.5 mg once weekly for 4 weeks. Next, we will quickly come up with a lifestyle habit goal for the next 4 weeks. You will make the choice of what this will be. Now we can add a healthy food, take away an unhealthy food you may be having a bit too much of, increase exercise of some kind, or discuss adding a stress-reducing activity during the week. What would you like to work on?

M: I would like to add a healthy food.

Dr. C: Great. Now let's choose between either adding a cup of berries or dark leafy greens or flaxseed. What do you want to do?

M: I like the idea of berries. I really have not been doing that too much.

Dr. C: Perfect. One of the healthiest foods on the planet for sure. This will impact health in several different ways. Now let's use the SMART technique to help make this goal successful. How many times a week will you have a cup of berries? I would suggest 4–5, but we can start anywhere that you think is realistic.

M: I can do 3.

Dr. C: Three it is. So, a cup of berries. And this can be blueberries, strawberries, blackberries, or raspberries. Three times a week for the next 4 weeks is our goal. Does that sound ok to you?

M: Yes, it does.

Dr. C: When do you think you would have this cup of berries during the day? Such as with breakfast or after dinner to make it like a dessert? I ask, because, the more specific we make the goal, the higher the chance of success.

M: I will add a cup of blueberries, as they are my favorite berries on Monday, Wednesday, and Fridays for breakfast.

Dr. C: Love the specific goal you just made. Well done. I will see you again in 6 weeks. Anything else for me today?

M: I am all good Dr. Chatterjee. Thank you.

NOTES

1 Ramage et al. *Applied Physiology, Nutrition and Metabolism* (2014). PMID: 24383502

2 Burke et al. *Journal of the American Dietetic Association* (2011). PMID: 21185970

3 Wing et al. *Obesity* (2021). PMID: 33988896

4 Oettingen et al. *Social and Personality Psychology Compass* (2016). DOI: 10.1111/spc3.12271

5 Armstrong et al. *Obesity Reviews* (2011). PMID: 21692966

6 Makin et al. *Clinical Obesity* (2021). PMID: 33955152

7 Seligman et al. *American Psychologist* (2000). PMID: 11392865

8 Richards et al. *Eating and Weight Disorders* (2021). PMID: 32424560

9 Arble et al. *Obesity* (2009). PMID: 19730426

10 Wang et al. *Obesity Reviews* (2014). PMID: 24888416

11 Wang et al. *European Heart Journal* (2021). PMID: 34374755

12 Brum et al. *Diabetology and Metabolic syndrome* (2020). PMID: 32064002

13 Strohmaier et al. *Current Diabetes Reports* (2018). PMID: 30343445

Index

Note: *Italic* page numbers refer to figures.

Printed in the United States
by Baker & Taylor Publisher Services